THE HEART DISEASE
REFERENCE BOOK

THE HEART DISEASE REFERENCE BOOK

Direct and clear answers to everyone's questions

Alan Mackintosh MA, MD, MRCP

Consultant Cardiologist
St. James's University Hospital & Killingbeck Hospital,
Leeds

Harper & Row, Publishers
London

Cambridge
Hagerstown
Philadelphia
New York

San Francisco
Mexico City
São Paulo
Sydney

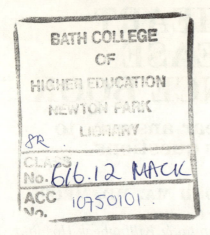
First published 1984

Harper and Row Ltd
28 Tavistock Street
London WC2E 7PN

British Library Cataloguing in Publication Data

Mackintosh, Alan
  The heart disease reference book.
  1. Heart — Diseases
  I. Title
  616.1'2   RC681

ISBN 0-06-318297-1

Typeset by Gedset Limited, Cheltenham
Printed and bound by Butler and Tanner Ltd, Frome and London

Contents

Preface

Books on heart disease abound. Any self-respecting medical bookshop will have a whole section devoted to the topic. Alternatively a number of simple books are available for sale to the general public: particular subjects in heart disease are covered by many free booklets and pamphlets. Information on the heart is widely available in many publications from Britain and America. English is also the international language of medicine, and heart books from other European countries may be published in English rather than the local language.

So why threaten to overburden readers with yet another book on the subject? Existing publications largely fall into two groups. Those in the first group for the general public, are limited in scope. They are either kept very simple and so provide little real information, or they are designed to propagate the author's own hobby-horse — 'do this and all will be well'. They deal almost exclusively with one form of heart disease, coronary artery disease, and the emphasis is on prevention. An idealized picture of personal and medical success emerges. People are not fooled that easily. They know that heart disease cannot be prevented in the sense of abolishing it; though the risk can be reduced. They are also aware, often from direct experience with a relative, that some forms of heart disease can prove fatal, in spite of the best efforts of doctors. These books for the general public fulfil a useful role in spreading information, but they fail to provide a full account of heart disease.

But when an interested reader turns to the second group of books, the medical publications, he is liable to suffer an acute attack of scientific indigestion. Those written for medical students and doctors assume a great deal of basic knowledge in anatomy and physiology. Not many people will have the time for the two-year course required in these subjects! The books for nurses, radiographers, and other paramedical professionals are more accessible, but they tend to concentrate on particular aspects useful to these health service staff. They are also rather dry, being written largely for the purpose of passing examinations.

This book hopes to provide a full account of heart disease for the many people who are not doctors, but who want to know about the problems of this important organ. They may have heart disease themselves or know a friend or a relative who has. They could be working in a job, such as a hospital administrator, medical journalist or ambulanceman, which would be helped by access to this information. They may already have some knowledge as part of their training for nursing or a paramedical profession, but are seeking a fuller picture. They might just be curious and need something to read on the train.

This book is not a textbook. It is also not trying to have the last word on the many controversial topics that are encountered in this field. The aim is not only to provide information, but also some of the flavour of heart disease in the late twentieth century. Which topics do doctors argue about? Why are governments slow to support preventative measures? Is the high cost of heart surgery justifiable? Should we really be worrying about the fats in our diet? This book should be comprehensible to anybody with a reasonable degree of general education. No specialist knowledge is assumed, but to avoid repetition some of the common terms are explained in the glossary rather than the main text. Most forms of heart disease are mentioned somewhere, though the rarer ones may only get a line or two.

Such is the aim of the book, but what is the aim of the author? After reading this book, some people should know more about heart disease. It is by far the commonest fatal illness in the westernized world; but also an illness that is partly preventable and can require expensive forms of treatment. Doctors no longer work in isolation from social and economic pressures — if they ever did.

The public needs to know what is going on, so that it can, through its representatives, define priorities and get the sort of Health Service it wants. Medicine is too important to be left to doctors alone.

Alan Mackintosh
1984

Glossary

Medical terminology and spelling vary from country to country. In this book British usage has been adhered to. Most drugs are referred to by at least two names. The one beginning with a small letter (propranolol) is the official non-proprietary name. Those starting with a capital letter (Inderal) are pharmaceutical company names. A drug has a single non-proprietary name, but may have more than one pharmaceutical company name, if several companies are marketing it. Only the commoner names can be given.

In this glossary some of the frequently used terms are explained; others can be found in the index. The descriptions apply particularly to heart disease. Some of the words may change their meanings when used in other fields.

angina
Chest pain, produced by the heart, which characteristically comes on with exercise or emotion and is relieved by rest.

aorta
Single main artery which leaves the heart. Divides into many smaller arteries.

arrhythmia
Abnormal heart rhythm.

artery
One of the several thick-walled, pulsating, blood vessels which take the blood from the heart to the lungs or the rest of the body.

atria
The two (right and left) collecting chambers of the heart. The veins drain into them and they in turn pass the blood into the main pumping chambers, the ventricles.

bradycardia
Abnormal slow heart rhythm.

calcify
Deposition of calcium; often in a heart valve.

capillary
Minute vessels connecting the arteries to the veins. In the capillaries the oxygen and other essential substances leave the blood, while carbon dioxide and waste products are taken up.

carbon dioxide
An end-product of cell biochemistry. It is removed by the blood and then blown off from the lungs.

cardiac
An adjective for anything to do with the heart, e.g. cardiac pain, cardiac ward.

catecholamines
A type of hormone. Hormones are messenger chemicals which circulate in the blood and control various bodily functions. Catecholamines are particularly involved in the reponse to acute stress.

cell
The basic 'building block' of all organs, usually only a few thousandths of a millimetre in diameter.

congenital
Adjective applied to defects which are present at birth.

coronary arteries
Arteries supplying the heart muscle itself. 'Coronary' is applied to anything related to these arteries, e.g. coronary thrombosis. 'A coronary' is a casual term for a myocardial infarction (see below).

cusp
The pulmonary and aortic valves are each made up of three cusps.

diastole
The period during each heart beat when the ventricles are relaxed and filling with blood from the atria. It coincides with the minimum (hence diastolic) blood pressure.

echocardiogram
An image of parts of the heart obtained with special sound waves.

electrocardiogram (ECG)
A recording of the amplified electrical signals from the heart.

electrode
An electrical contact with the body. For an electrocardiogram, or cardiac monitoring in a coronary care unit, it is used to record electricity. As part of a pacemaker 'wire' its purpose is to convey electricity to the heart muscle for stimulation.

emboli
Solid or gaseous matter, such as a clot or air, which travels in the blood stream and can obstruct an artery.

heart attack
An ill-defined term. In this book other, more specific, descriptions such as myocardial infarction, are preferred.

hormone
Messenger chemical circulating in the blood.

hyperlipidaemia
Raised blood fats.

hypertension
Elevated blood pressure

hypertrophy
Progressive enlargement, often referring to heart muscle - ventricular hypertrophy.

incompetence
In heart disease it commonly alludes to a leaking heart valve, e.g. mitral incompetence.

infarction
Permanent damage to cells secondary to a period of inadequ-

ate blood supply. In a myocardial infarction some heart muscle cells are destroyed and replaced by a scar.

ischaemia
Disordered function due to a shortage of oxygenated blood. It is often temporary: the cells recover once a normal supply is restored. If not, infarction follows.

leaflet
Component of the mitral and tricuspid valves. The mitral valve has two leaflets and the tricuspid has three.

left heart
Left atrium and left ventricle.

lipids
Fats in the blood

myocardium
Heart muscle, hence 'myocardial infarction'.

oedema
Abnormal accumulation of fluid outside the blood vessels. Commonly in the lungs (pulmonary oedema) or at the ankles.

pulmonary
Adjective for anything related to the lungs.

right heart
Right atrium and right ventricle.

Risk factor
Personal characteristic associated with an increased risk of an illness, usually coronary artery disease.

stenosis
An abnormal obstruction to blood flow, especially a narrowed heart valve, e.g. mitral stenosis.

systemic
Part of the circulation to the body as opposed to the pulmonary circulation to the lungs.

systole
Period of ventricular contraction and ejection of blood from

the heart. Systolic (blood) pressure is the maximum blood pressure.

tachycardia
 Abnormal fast heart rhythm.

thrombosis
 Blood clotting in an artery or vein.

valve
 Venous valves prevent blood flowing backwards in the veins. The four heart valves keep the blood moving in the correct direction through the heart. When healthy they prevent back flow without obstructing forward movement

Valve	*Orifice*	
tricuspid	right atrium ⟶	right ventricle
pulmonary	right ventricle ⟶	pulmonary artery
mitral	left atrium ⟶	left ventricle
aortic	left ventricle ⟶	aorta

veins
 Low-pressure blood vessels which collect the blood from the body or lungs and return it to the heart.

ventricles
 The two (right and left) main pumping chambers of the heart.

1

The problem of heart disease

The heart is an exceedingly important piece of muscle and fibre. In mechanical terms the heart is no more than a well-designed pump; but in emotional terms it is a lot more than this. The heart has a central role in life, not just in disease. Few people can view their own heart as just being a tough piece of muscle. The hearts of others can be thought of in these dispassionate terms, but not your own.

The heart is important as the organ that pumps the blood to the rest of the body. The organs are entirely dependent on it. If the heart stops beating they will soon lose their function and become irreversibly damaged. The first organ to be affected is the brain; the patient is unconscious within a few seconds of the heart stopping. More commonly, the organs may be chronically starved of blood by a defective heart. They do not function well and the patient feels tired and listless. This is in addition to the more specific heart symptoms of pain and breathlessness.

The pattern of disease changes over the years. In the fourteenth century the Black Death (plague) killed about a quarter of the population of England. Two hundred years later Europeans seemed to be at the mercy of syphilis, fresh from the recently discovered continent of America. Cholera was a scourge in the nineteenth century until sewers and a good water supply prevented its easy transmission from person to person. In the second half of the twentieth century heart disease, that is coronary artery disease, is the major epidemic in the developed world. About four million people in Britain have some form of heart disease. The exact number is unknown as no system exists for the registration of such a common illness. About half of all men have had some heart trouble by the age of 65. A long bus queue will normally contain at least one person with a diseased heart, though he or she may not have told any friends about it. Three times as many working days are lost from heart disease than are lost from industrial disputes.

But heart disease is more than just a common problem; colds and chest infections are common too. Heart disease can be fatal and it is easily the commonest cause of death in Britain. Approximately 200,000 people die from it each year, twice the death rate from all types of cancer. The vast majority of these heart disease deaths are due to coronary artery disease. Many of the victims are elderly, but deaths from heart disease can occur at any age, including the first day of life. In a few countries such as the United States, the number of deaths is falling sharply, in many like Britain it is constant or falling slightly, and in some it is increasing.

As the function of the heart can be easily imagined and because heart disease may be fatal, the patient will rarely think of his problem in a straighforward manner. Emotions and heart disease become closely linked. In some patients it may take the form of an initial denial that their symptoms are anything to do with the heart: doctors are particularly good at this when they develop heart symptoms. Others go to the opposite extreme of severe anxiety for a minor problem. Such anxiety will by itself make the patient ill. It can produce tiredness, palpitations, and difficulty in breathing, which in turn may convince the patient that the heart disease is more severe than the doctor has indicated. Most doctors become quite adept at sorting out the heart symptoms from the anxiety symptoms. They have to be, as this combination will often be encountered.

More tragic is the individual who is convinced that his healthy heart is diseased. The protean symptoms of some heart problems can be mimicked by a wide variety of other diseases and it can be difficult from just the patient's story and physical examination to decide at once whether the heart is healthy or not. A doctor may be hesitant to come to a definite conclusion at first. Words like 'might have heart disease' can be misconstrued as a definite diagnosis of heart trouble, allowing a long-term misconception to develop. In a strange fashion it can be comforting to have heart disease as a generally accepted explanation for a symptom such as chest pain. The patient knows where he stands and sympathy is automatic. Doctors dealing with heart disease know how a patient's face may droop with disappointment when he is told that the pain is not coming from his heart.

So heart disease is rarely a simple technical problem of dealing with a disordered pump. The patient's previous experiences, current emotions, and future expectations are intimately tied up with it. For the doctor every word must be picked with care. The patient must try to assimilate any advice, concentrating on what is said and resisting his own embellishments.

2

The healthy heart

'...the blood in the animal body is impelled in a circle, and
is in a state of ceaseless motion; this is the act or function
which the heart performs by means of its pulse; and it is the
sole and only end of the motion and contraction of the
heart.'

William Harvey, 1628

William Harvey was the first person to appreciate the correct
function of the heart and blood vessels. He realized over
three hundred years ago that the heart only has one action
— pumping blood around the body. But this task has to be
performed once or twice per second for 70 years or more.
Cessation of the circulation will produce symptoms within a
few seconds and death within minutes. The heart must be
reliable. It must also be *adaptable* to the changing needs of
the body. During exercise the body may require a six-fold
increase in blood flow. The heart has to provide the right
quantity of blood or the muscles cannot work efficiently.
Remarkably, the heart responds to the increased demand
within a few beats. As a sprinter bursts from his starting
blocks, the heart will adapt almost immediately. No other
organ in the body has such continuous demands placed upon
it.

Structure

The healthy heart is mostly muscle with some fibrous elements, nerves, and blood vessels, weighing in all about 300 grams (10 ounces). The type of muscle is unique to the heart; other muscles do not have to contract and relax continously. The heart is at the front of the chest, in the centre and over to the left (Figure 2.1). Anatomically, left and right refer to the position as seen from the back of the subject. The pulsation in the left side of the chest, that can sometimes be felt or seen, represents the left-hand border of the heart; the rest of it is more central. The position of this pulsation has led to the misconception that all of the heart is in the left side of the chest. Also the conventional picture of a heart as found on a Valentine card or carved on a tree does not portray the human heart. Its size and shape are similar to the clenched fist of a large right hand, with the back of the hand facing forward and the knuckles pointing down.

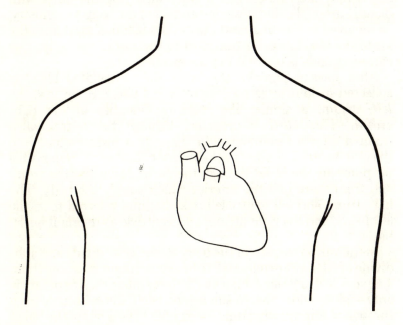

Figure 2.1. The position of the heart

The heart functions as two separate pumps, supplying the two systems of blood vessels (circulations) in the body (Figure 2.2). One circulation supplies the lungs (pulmonary circulation) and the other meets the needs of the rest of the body (systemic circulation). The blood coming back to the heart from the rest of the body collects in a thin-walled, low-pressure, cavity known as the right atrium, which is named after a supposed resemblance to the central court of an ancient Roman house. The blood, which is low in oxygen, passes through the tricuspid valve into a thicker-walled pumping chamber called the right ventricle. Three mobile structures (leaflets) make up the tricuspid valve and give it a name. The right ventricle pumps the blood into the pulmonary artery. The pumping action closes the triscupid valve preventing blood flow backwards into the right atrium. Similarly a pulmonary valve prevents blood regurgitating back into the right ventricle from the pulmonary artery. This vessel splits into two main arteries which in turn divide and sub-divide like branches of a tree, supplying the lungs with blood, Carbon dioxide, a waste-product of the body's chemistry, is removed in the lungs and the oxygen is transferred from the air to the blood cells for transport to the rest of the body. The carbon dioxide is blown off in the exhaled air.

After passing through the lungs the oxygenated blood is collected in four large pulmonary veins which drain into the *left* atrium, a similar low-pressure chamber to the right atrium. The blood is propelled through the mitral valve (named after a resemblance in shape to a bishop's hat) into the *left* ventricle. This thick-walled chamber is responsible for pumping the blood through the aortic valve into the aorta and from there into the arteries which supply the body. The left atrium and left ventricle are sometimes referred to as the left heart, and the right atrium and ventricle as the right heart. heart.

In the various organs of the body the arteries divide and sub-divide until they are too small to be seen without magnification. The smallest arteries connect with the capillaries. A capillary is only slightly wider than a single blood cell; the cells have to go through in line allowing time for oxygen to flow out of the blood and waste products, such as carbon dioxide, to diffuse in. At the

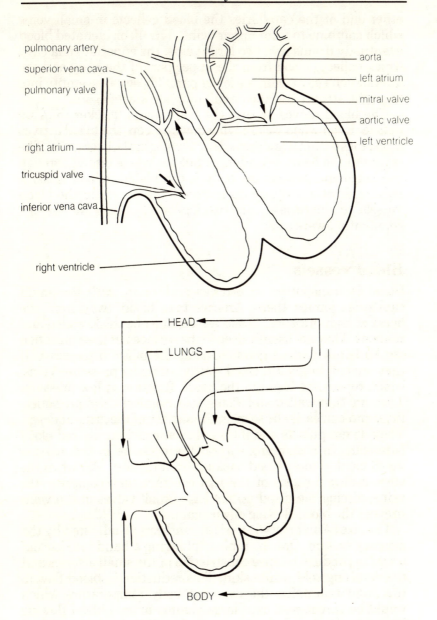

pulmonary artery
superior vena cava
pulmonary valve

aorta
left atrium
mitral valve
aortic valve
left ventricle

right atrium

tricuspid valve

inferior vena cava

right ventricle

HEAD
LUNGS

BODY

Figure 2.2. The structure of the heart and the circulation of blood in the body

other end of the capillaries the blood collects in small veins which combine to form bigger veins. The deoxygenated blood eventually drains into two large veins, the superior vena cava which collects blood from the upper part of the body and the inferior vena cava from the lower part. These cavae empty into the right atrium and the circuit of blood starts again.

The blood moves around the body much quicker than we realize. Even when we are lying down asleep, the blood arrives at the toes within a few seconds of leaving the left ventricle. The return to the heart takes longer but the whole circuit through the lungs and around the body is completed in well under a minute. Fortunately we do not have the nerves in the blood vessels to appreciate this rushing of blood, so we are not constantly aware of it.

Blood vessels

Blood is transported in arteries and veins, with the small capillaries joining them. Arteries take blood away from the heart at high pressure. These vessels must be thick-walled and resilient. They are usually deep to the surface but their pulsation can be felt at various points such as the pulse in the wrist. If they are cut, bright red blood spurts out under pressure. Veins, which return the blood to the heart, function at low pressure. They are thin-walled and distensible. Some of them are superficial and can easily be seen on the surface of the arms and legs. They do not pulsate and if they are damaged purply-red blood oozes out. In a standing subject the pressure in the veins is insufficient to force blood back up from the feet. But when the surrounding muscles of the legs contract they compress the veins, forcing the blood up the legs. Small valves in the veins prevent the blood flowing down again.

The size of an artery is variable and can be adjusted by the nervous system. One example is plunging a hand into icecold water to produce intense constriction of the small arteries and the resulting cold, white skin. This reduction in blood flow to the hand maintains the constant body temperature which would be threatened by a large volume of cold blood flowing back from the hand. Arteries may also dilate to promote blood flow to an organ; one example is the stomach after a meal.

Blood pressure

The pressure in the arteries rises and falls as the heart pumps. The maximum pressure is referred to as the systolic pressure as it is produced by ventricular contraction (systole). A typical systolic pressure would be 140 millimetres of mercury in a systemic artery and 30 millimetres in the pulmonary artery. The minimum pressure corresponds to ventricular relaxation (diastole) and is called the diastolic pressure. Typical values might be 80 millimetres of mercury in a systemic artery and 15 millimetres in the pulmonary artery. For those who are not familiar with pressure measurements, 15 millimetres of mercury means that the pressure would just support a column of mercury 15 millimetres high. The maximum and minimum pressures in a systemic artery are often combined (for example 140/80) and referred to as the blood pressure. High blood pressure (hypertension) will be discussed in a later chapter.

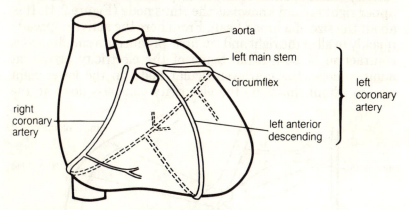

Figure 2.3. The coronary arteries

Coronary arteries

Disease of the arteries which supply the heart muscle itself (coronary arteries) is the commonest form of heart disease in the developed world; so these arteries are particularly important. Like any muscle, heart muscle needs a reliable blood supply to function satisfactorily. Two coronary arteries branch off the aorta just as it leaves the heart (Figure 2.3) and then run across the outside of the heart. The left coronary artery has a short main stem and soon divides into the circumflex and left anterior descending arteries. The right coronary artery continues as a single vessel. The division of the left coronary artery produces a total of three vessels to supply blood to the heart muscle. Doctors talk about one, two, or three vessel disease to indicate the extent of any arterial damage. As in other organs the arteries divide and sub-divide to supply the minute capillaries, where the exchange of gases and removal of waste products takes place. Most of the veins connect with one large vein, the coronary sinus, at the back of the heart. The coronary sinus returns the deoxygenated blood to the right atrium.

Heart rhythm

Contraction of the heart muscle is triggered by small electric currents of less than a hundredth of a Volt. This electrical activity starts spontaneously in a specialized structure in the upper right atrium known as the sinus node (Figure 2.4). It is about the size of a broad bean. From here the activity spreads quickly to all of the right and left atria producing a simultaneous contraction of both atria. Some of the electricity arrives at another node, the antrioventricular node, in the lower right atrium. From this node the electricity can pass down to the

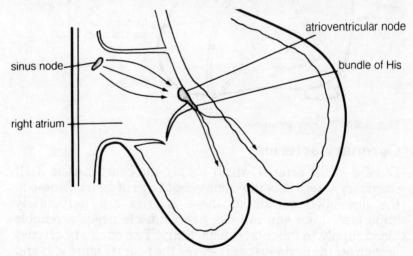

Figure 2.4. Electrical activity in a heart beat

ventricles using an electrical bridge known as the Bundle of His, which is named after the man who first described it. Conducting fibres spread out from the lower end of the Bundle of His to activate both ventricles and time must be allowed for this to occur before ventricular contraction. So an important requirement for efficient pumping is a delay between atrial and ventricular activation. The electrical signals are retarded for about a tenth of a second in the antrioventricular node. When added to the time taken for the electricity to spread into the ventricles this produces a total interval of about two tenths of a second between atrial and ventricular contraction.

Control of the heart

The heart is able to increase its output within a few seconds of the onset of exercise or other circulatory demands. It can do this by increasing the heart rate or by adjusting the volume of blood pumped by each beat.

The heart rate is largely under the control of the body's nervous system. As we have seen, the timing of the heart beat is controlled by the sinus node in the right atrium which discharges an electrical signal to the rest of the heart. The node can function independently but it is well supplied with nerves which slow down (known as parasympathetic nerves) or speed up (sympathetic nerves) the discharge rate. The rate is also influenced by hormones which are circulating chemicals in the blood stream. The best known hormone is adrenaline. The speed of the heart is the sum of these various influences. The node can function satisfactorily if the nerves are blocked but it loses its ability to perform a rapid rate change. The healthy heart speeds up as soon as exercise is started.

Although a rise in the heart rate is the major mechanism for augmenting the output of the healthy heart, the volume pumped with each beat can also be increased. The volume of blood returning to the heart becomes larger with exercise. An important property of the heart muscle is that stretching of the muscle fibres by the increased volume of blood makes the muscle contract more forcibly. So the right ventricle can eject this increased volume of blood through the lung vessels into the left atrium. The same mechanism ensures that the increased volume is quicklly pumped to the body be the left ventrical.

Conclusion

For most of us the heart works normally for decades. Even if problems occur the heart can often overcome them by suitable adaptations without the subject being aware of any disease. But certain parts of the heart, such as the valves, electrical conduction system, or coronary arteries are more crucial and damage may result in illness. This book is concerned with heart disease but we should not forget the heart's remarkable ability to pump continously for a whole lifetime.

3

Symptoms, diagnosis, and investigations

Accurate diagnosis is the essential first step in the management of heart disease. Does the patient have heart disease? What type is it? How severe is it? The starting point is the symptoms that are troubling the patient. Fortunately for the doctor, heart disease only produces a small range of symptoms. So the initial approach does not vary much. The techniques used to get the correct diagnosis will be described in this chapter. The details of different types of heart disease will be dealt with later.

Arriving at a diagnosis consists of three stages. The first is the patient's *symptoms*; what does he complain about? The second is the examination to detect any *signs* of heart disease. The last part is any *investigations* that are needed to confirm the diagnosis or assess the severity of the disorder. In many patients all necessary information is obtained from the first two stages, so investigations are not required.

Pain

This is the symptom that produces most anxiety. Heart pain is usually, but not always, felt in the chest. Chest pains are common, as are stomach aches, backaches, headaches and other pains. But more attention is always paid to chest pain than to other pains because heart disease is a possible cause. Any anxiety will magnify the pain. Although chest pain occurs in some forms of heart disease, it can be produced by many other things. The majority of pains in the chest are nothing to do with the heart.

Heart pain is commonly felt in the middle of the chest and may seem to spread across the chest, down the arms, or up into the neck and jaw (Figure 3.1). Examples have been described of the pain being felt everywhere from the nose to the upper thighs, but the vast majority of heart pains are felt in the chest. The pain has a diffuse feel to it and cannot be localized precisely, as can the pain from a superficial cut or bruise. The pain is commonly described as tight, crushing, or pressure. Pain that is sharp, stabbing, or like a pin is unlikely to come from the heart. Pure heart pain is not affected by breathing but pain from the tissues around the heart (p.126) can be made worse by a deep breath. Heart pain can be very severe, making the patient look unwell, pale and sweaty.

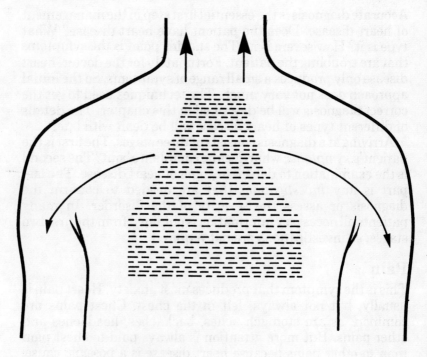

Figure 3.1. Site of heart pain

What causes heart pain?

The pain is produced by an imbalance between the oxygen availability and the oxygen requirement of the heart muscles. If insufficient oxygen gets through to the muscle, pain-producing chemicals are formed. Oxygen is carried by blood so one cause of the pain is obstruction of blood flow in the coronary arteries. On the other hand the blood flow can be normal but the heart muscle has increased in thickness, resulting in more oxygen being needed; the blood flow cannot cope with the extra demand. An example of this effect would be the thickened heart muscle that is necessary to force the blood through an obstructed aortic valve (p.98).

Why is the pain felt in the middle of the chest when much of the heart is on the left side?

The nerves that record pain from the heart are different from those that deal with the skin and chest wall. The heart nerves cannot localize a pain precisely, so it is felt felt over a wide area. In the early stage of its development the heart is a symmetrical, midline, structure. The nerves still seem to work on this basis although the heart later becomes more leftsided. The arms develop from the same region as the heart so the pain is often felt in the arms as well.

Can heart pain be felt in the left side of the chest?

Yes, but the middle is a more common site. To put it the other way round, most leftsided chest pains, particularly if they are felt at one point, come from the muscles and joints of the chest wall.

Can the pain be felt in the back?

Yes, but it is unusual for heart pain to be felt just in the back.

Why does heart pain tend to come and go, rarely persisting for long periods?

Pain that occurs with exertion makes the patient stop and rest. The oxygen requirements are then reduced and the pain is relieved. This is the typical pattern for *angina*. Pain that occurs at rest following an acute obstruction of a coronary artery may persist for several hours. An oxygen shortage over this period will kill heart muscle cells. This is known as an *infarction*. Dead cells no longer require oxygen and the pain will go. Angina and infarction will be described in more detail in Chapter 4.

Breathlessness

The breathlessness of heart disease is usually produced by excess fluid in the lungs — pulmonary oedema. The oedema is produced by an inability of the left ventricle to pump enough blood out of the heart — left heart failure. As a result the pressure in the left atrium rises, increasing the pressure in the lung veins that feed into it. This pressure forces some of the fluid in the blood out of the lung vessels and into the lung itself. The solid part of the blood, particularly the corpuscles that give the blood its red colour, are kept in the vessels. The excess fluid in the lungs makes them stiffer and increases the work of breathing. In addition it reduces the movement of gases in and out of the blood stream which means that the patient has to breathe faster to oxygenate the blood. In severe cases frothy fluid may be coughed up.

Why is the breathlessness worse on exercise and better with rest?

With exercise the output of the heart rises to provide more oxygen and other substances to the muscles. If left heart failure is present the left ventricle will find it more difficult to pump the increased volume of blood arriving from the right heart. The left atrial pressure will rise further, forcing more fluid into the lung tissue.

Why is breathlessness often brought on by lying down flat?

The veins, the blood vessels that drain the blood into the heart, are thin-walled, distensible, structures. On sitting or standing some of the blood pools in the veins of the legs and pelvis. If the patient then lies down, the pooled blood returns to the heart and is quickly pumped to the lungs, driving more fluid out into the lung tissue. Many patients with left heart failure prefer to sleep propped up on several pillows or even sitting in a chair.

Why do such patients often wake up breathless in the middle of the night?

They slip down the bed and wake up as the fluid accumulates in the lungs. Sitting up soon relieves the symptoms.

Ankle Swelling

As we have just seen, if the left heart fails fluid accumulates in the lungs. In a similar fashion, if the right heart fails the pressure rises in the veins of the body and fluid is forced out. This fluid (oedema) collects in the lowest part of the body where the venous pressure is highest — the ankles in the average ambulant patient. Sometimes the fluid is also found inside the abdomen.

Although ankle swelling can occur in heart failure the vast majority of swollen ankles are nothing to do with the heart. Some fluid around the ankles is common after standing, especially in women, and it is not by itself a sign of heart disease.

How does the doctor decide that ankle swelling is produced by heart disease?

He looks for other signs of excess blood in the veins. Because the right heart is not pumping blood to the lungs fast enough, the veins are distended. The veins on the side of the neck are the best guide. They normally empty on sitting up but remain full if the venous pressure is raised.

Can a swollen face be due to heart failure?

Only under very exceptional circumstances when the face is lower than the rest of the body for a prolonged period. With normal standing, sitting or lying positions the fluid would collect elsewhere.

Malaise

A reduced output of blood from the heart also produces non-specific symptoms of tiredness, listlessness, and lack of energy. They can be grouped together under the term 'malaise'. The underlying problem is the heart's inability to deliver enough blood to the muscles. In a sense the muscles slow down to avoid outstripping their blood supply

Malaise is a common complaint. Is it often secondary to heart disease?

The vast majority of people who complain of it will not have heart disease. On the other hand a few people with heart disease will not notice it because the onset was very gradual or they just feel they are getting old. A comparison with other people of a similar age can be very useful.

Could a person whose only complaint is tiredness have heart disease?

This is possible but unlikely. Tiredness produced by heart disease will usually be accompanied by another symptom such as chest pain or breathlessness. Tiredness as the sole symptom is unusual.

Palpitations

Awareness of the heart beating regularly at a normal speed is not a symptom of heart disease. We are normally unaware of the heart's action, but some of us can feel the beats at times. Palpitations is a term reserved for awareness of rapid beating. But a fast heart does not have to be abnormal. Its speed varies with activity and emotion. At rest the heart beats between 50 and 110 times a minutes. A rate of 140 beats per minute would be normal during exercise or acute anxiety, but abnormal while sitting quietly. The heart rate can change within seconds, especially in the young. Worry about how fast the heart is beating is enough, by itself, to increase the rate above 100 per minute in some people.

What produces palpitations?

The abnormal, fast heart beat may only be a sign that the diseased heart is working harder to maintain the blood flow round the body. But the palpitations can be due to an abnormal *rhythm.* Part of the heart starts beating rapidly and drives the rest of the heart at a faster speed. Using the example of a motor car, it is as if the engine is working normally but the ignition is driving it at the wrong speed.

Are palpitations regular or irregular?

They can be either. Irregular palpitations are less likely to be produced by anxiety and so are more likely to be a symptom of heart disease.

How are palpitations produced by heart disease distinguished from those secondary to anxiety?

It can be difficult. Palpitations produced by abnormal rhythms tend to come on suddenly and stop suddenly; anxiety produces a more gradual onset and disappearance. The circumstances when the rapid beating starts can be helpful. Other evidence of heart disease is sought to solve the problem. Tests may be necessary.

Why do patients feel tired during palpitations produced by heart disease?

The rhythm may be too fast to allow sufficient time for the heart to empty and fill fully with each beat. This will reduce the cardiac output and produce the malaise described earlier.

Why are palpitations sometimes accompanied by chest pain?

The faster rate increases the oxygen requirements of the heart muscle. As described earlier, if the blood flow to the heart muscle cannot keep pace with oxygen demands pain is felt. Palpitations only produce this effect if the heart is diseased in some other way.

Dizziness and blackouts

Heart disease is one possible cause of these symptoms. If the heart beats too slowly or stops for a few seconds the organs are temporarily starved of blood. The brain is very sensitive to this oxygen shortage and its function is soon upset. Dizziness and unsteadiness can result, or even loss of consciousness if the shortage is more prolonged. So heart disease can be a cause of unexplained falls, especially in the elderly.

Can these symptoms be dangerous?

They can be, depending on the underlying heart disease. But the loss of consciousness is protective. Once the patient has fallen down the blood flows easily back to the heart through horizontal veins. This improves the output from the heart and in turn the blood flow to the brain increases.

How do these symptoms differ from faints?

Simple faints are not due to heart disease though they produce similar effect. A faint is due to blood pooling in the legs, often during prolonged standing. This reduces the amount of blood available to go to the brain. The subject falls down, immediately correcting the situation.

What is the duration of dizziness and blackouts due to heart disease?

They come and go quite suddenly, usually within a minute or two. The heart has several self-correcting mechanisms that limit the duration of these symptoms. If the dizziness or blackouts persist, they are unlikely to be produced by the heart.

In addition to asking about some or all of these symptoms, the doctor may want to know about the amount of activity undertaken at work or leisure, smoking habits, previous drug therapy, earlier medical examinations, and past illnesses and operations. He may enquire about heart disease in close relatives as some disorders run in families. After listening to the patient's story and asking the relevant questions he may have already completely ruled out heart disease, making further assessment unnecessary. If not, he will start the examination.

Examination

The next stage in arriving at a diagnosis is to examine the body so that signs of heart disease can be looked at, felt, or heard. If the diagnosis is already clear from the description of the symptoms the examination may be brief. If considerable doubt exists it may be painstaking and repeated. The heart is normally examined with the patient propped up at about 45°. This is partly because it is comfortable for both patient and doctor, and partly because it enables the venous pressure in the neck veins to be seen clearly.

Why does the doctor stand on the patient's right side during the examination?

Most doctors, like everybody else, are right-handed, so examination is easier from that side. Also the heart is on the left of the chest and it can be best felt from the other side.

Why are the eyes examined with an instrument when the problem is heart disease?

The front of the eye is transparent, so the blood vessels inside the eye can be seen with a magnifying instrument (ophthalmo-scope). Any damage to the eye blood vessels is a guide to the state of the similar heart blood vessels.

What is the doctor listening for with his stethoscope?

He can hear the sounds of the heart valves closing — the familiar 'lub-dub' sound popular on the sound track of suspense and horror films. The diseased heart may produce additional sounds, particularly the noises (murmurs) prod-uced by the disordered valves or abnormal holes in the heart muscle. With a very talkative patient it is also an opportunity for a few seconds of uninterrupted thought.

Why does the doctor examine other parts of the body even when the problem is heart disease?

Heart disease affects other organs. For example, the venous engorgement of heart failure can increase the size of the liver. The doctor is also trying to exclude other diseases as a cause of the symptoms.

Investigations

In general practice the symptoms and examination will provide an accurate diagnosis most of the time. But more complex problems, particularly those referred to hospital, often require additional tests.

The number of tests performed will vary from patient to patient. The heart can be investigated in great detail if necessary. But such tests are time consuming, expensive, and sometimes uncomfortable.

The investigations have to be used with discretion, depending on the circumstances. In general the main indications are either to establish a diagnosis which is still uncertain or to clarify the severity of the heart disease when a complex treatment, such as cardiac surgery, is being considered. The tests can also be used to monitor the effectiveness of treatment.

Chest X-ray

X-rays find the solid structure of the heart more difficult to penetrate than the airfilled lungs around it. So the heart shows up as a silhouette on the chest X-ray with lungs on either side (Figure 3.2). Abnormalities in the shape or size of this silhouette help in the diagnosis of heart disease. The appearance of the lungs can also be useful. Chest X-rays are taken in a standard way all over the world. An X-ray of the chest taken in London should be very similar to the one taken on the same patient in Tokyo.

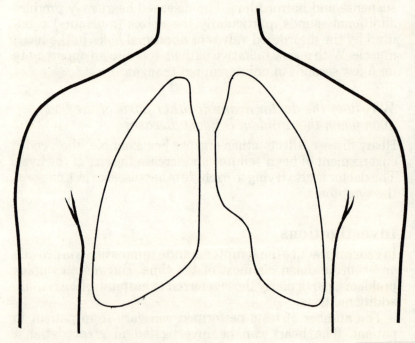

Figure 3.2. Heart silhouette on a chest X-ray

What can be learnt from the chest X-ray?

The size of the heart silhouette is an indicator of heart failure. The ventricles dilate and their walls thicken in an attempt to maintain cardiac output in chronic heart failure. This increases the overall size of the heart. A big heart can be detected by examination but the chest X-ray is more sensitive. This investigation can be used to monitor the progress of heart failure. Increasing heart size suggests that it is getting worse, while a diminution in size indicates improvement. The appearance of the lungs is also helpful in the diagnosis of a failing left ventricle. The fluid (oedema) that is pushed out of the blood vessels by rising pressure can be seen in the lungs on X-ray.

Apart from the overall size, an abnormal shape of the heart silhouette can have diagnostic value. Enlargement of the atria can be detected in this way. The shape of the healthy heart does not change much from the onset of adulthood to the beginning of old age. So an alteration from one chest X-ray to the next suggests some form of heart disease.

Sometimes a sideways (lateral) view will be taken as well as the normal chest X-ray. This will provide a different silhouette of the heart for diagnosis. It is also a good view for seeing calcium inside the heart. Diseased heart valves sometimes calcify in later life.

Although the chest X-ray is an important investigation it does have limitations. In most cases it will only reveal the outline of the heart — a silhouette, not a detailed portrait. More complex techniques (see below) are needed to visualize the structure inside the heart.

Electrocardiogram (ECG)

An electrocardiogram is a recording of small electrical signals from within the heart. As we saw in Chapter 2, the heart beat is normally started by a small area of pacemaker tissue (sinus node) in the right atrium. The electrical activity spreads to the rest of the heart, triggering a coordinated contraction of the atria and ventricles. The signals are very small, in the region of one thousandth of a Volt (a torch battery often generates 1.5 Volts). So the electricity has to be amplified in an electrocardiograph.

The method of recording the standard, 12-lead, electrocardiogram is the same throughout the world. An electrode is fastened to each limb (Figure 3.3). Another electrode is in turn used to record from six different positions on the front of the chest. Sometimes six electrodes are applied to the chest rather than moving one to six positions. By connecting up different pairs of limb electrodes, six limb lead recordings and six chest lead recordings are made.

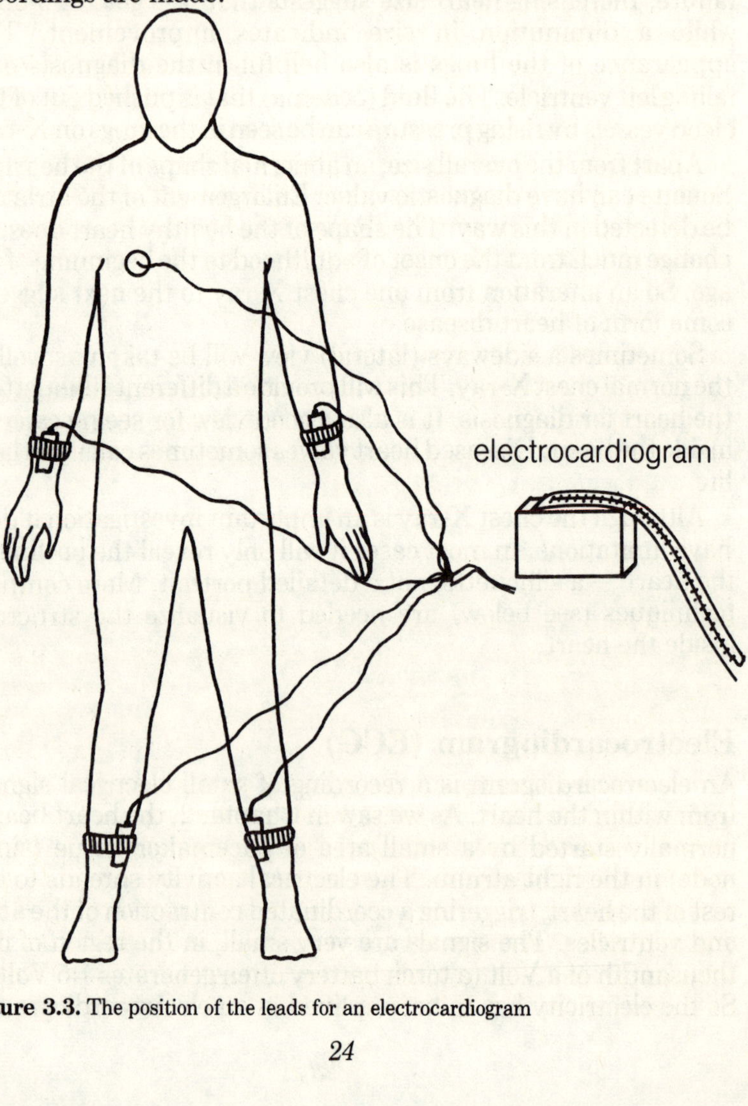

electrocardiogram

Figure 3.3. The position of the leads for an electrocardiogram

What can be learned from the electrocardiogram?

The rhythm of the heart can be illustrated. The examination may reveal whether the heart is going too fast or too slow, but an electrocardiogram is often needed to explain these abnormal rhythms. With a slow rhythm (bradycardia) the spread of electrical activity may have been interrupted. For a fast rhythm (tachycardia) part of the heart that usually waits to be excited may start to beat spontaneously, acting as an abnormal pacemaker for the rest of the heart.

The second type of information obtained is an impression of the state of health of the ventricular, and sometimes the atrial, muscle. Diseased heart muscle becomes electrically abnormal. For example, a shortage of oxygen in the ventricular muscle produces abnormalities in the recovery from contraction, which can be seen on the electrocardiogram. Dead heart tissue becomes electrically inexcitable; this may also alter the electrocardiogram.

How accurate is the electrocardiogram?

An electrocardiogram is mainly a supplementary investigation. By itself it will rarely give a clearcut answer. But taken in conjunction with the symptoms and examination it is very useful in confirming a suspected diagnosis.

Does a normal electrocardiogram rule out heart disease?

Unfortunately, no. It is possible, though not common, to have severe heart disease with a normal electrocardiogram. The disease can be confined to a small area of the heart so that it does not distort the electrical signals. Also the distinction between a normal and an abnormal electrocardiogram is not rigid. Most are definitely one or the other, but a few are in an area of uncertainty in between. Another reason for 'missing' heart disease is that the instrument is sensitive to heart disease at the front of the heart, close to the electrodes, but is less good for the back of the heart.

Although the electrocardiogram cannot by itself rule out heart disease, the doctor is often reassured by a normal tracing. If the doctor thinks that the patient's symptoms are unlikely to be due to heart disease, a normal electrocardiogram will support him in that conclusion. But if he is confident that the symptoms are produced by the heart a normal electrocardiogram will rarely make him change his mind.

Why are the electrocardiogram and chest X-ray often repeated?

Acute changes are more important than appearances that may have been present for years. The tests may need to be repeated to be certain that the abnormalities really are acute. The series of electrocardiograms that may be needed to confirm the diagnosis of a heart attack is an example of this. The tests may also be used to monitor the progress of the disease. A gradual increases in the heart size in a series of chest X-rays often indicates a steady deterioration in cardiac function.

Can taking the electrocardiogram hurt?

No. The electrocardiogram is only a recording of electricity coming out of the body. Nothing is put in.

Why is jelly smeared underneath the electrodes?

Dry skin is a poor conductor of electricity. Some old electrocardiographs used special wet pads. Nowadays a jelly containing a weak salt solution is used to improve conduction. The jelly is non-toxic and washes off easily.

Is the electrocardiogram changed by disease elsewhere in the body?

Yes, sometimes. Disturbances in the concentrations of minerals in the blood (particularly potassium) can affect the electrocardiogram. Also certain forms of head injuries can influence it; the reason for this interesting phenomenon is still uncertain. In some completely healthy people the electrocardiogram changes with excessively rapid breathing or severe emotion.

Exercise test

So far we have dealt with the electrocardiogram *at rest*. At times extra information can be gathered by recording the electrocardiogram during or immediately after exercise. This test is primarily a means of assessing the presence and extent of coronary artery disease. It is designed to stress the heart: 'stress test' is another name for it. The heart with narrowed coronary arteries may function normally at rest when the blood is pumped at a rate of about 3 litres a minute. But on exercise the cardiac output may rise to over 12 litres a minute. The diseased heart can no longer deal easily with this increased output and the electro-cardiogram becomes abnormal.

One type of exercise is repeatedly stepping up and down one or two small steps at a fixed rate. This technique requires little equipment but the amount of exercise performed is dependent on several variables, including the subject's weight. A better method of exercising is to peddle a stationary bicycle with a brake on the wheel to make it harder. The resistance of the brake is gradually increased. The amount of exercise can be measured, but the test is impossible in patients with arthritis or other problems in the legs. The most natural form of exercise test is to walk on a moving surface (Figure 3.4). The patient walks at the

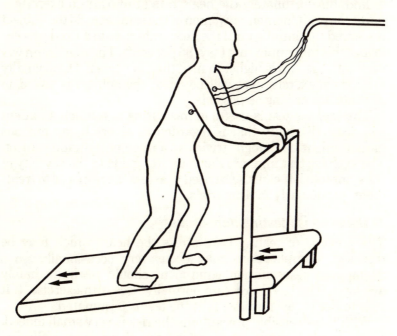

Figure 3.4. Exercise test with a moving surface

same speed as the surface moves so he stays in one place. The surface is gradually tilted and the speed increased to make walking progressively more difficult. This method is sometimes referred to as the 'treadmill test'. The term is misleading as the moving surface is driven by a motor, not by the patient.

Whatever the type of exercise, at least one lead of the electrocardiogram is monitored during exercise and the blood pressure is usually checked at intervals. A full electrocardiogram is done before and immediately after the exercise. Sometimes it is repeated a few minutes later.

When is exercise stopped?

In symptomatic patients the aim is to induce the symptoms and then stop. If no symptoms appear, the test is ended once a predetermined proportion of the maximum rate of exercise for a healthy subject has been achieved. This point might be difficult to find, but fortunately the heart rate at maximum exercise is fairly constant for men or women of the same age. So the subject is allowed to continue until the heart rate rises to a fixed percentage of this maximum rate (say, 85 per cent). The maximum will vary with age and is higher in men than in women. Occasionally a *maximal* exercise test will be used: the subject is asked to continue for as long as possible.

The exercise test is useful in measuring how much a patient can do. A disability that is regarded as severe by an anxious patient might be thought trivial by a more phlegmatic subject. The exercise test may provide a clearer guide to the severity of the symptoms. It can also be used to assess the response to treatment, particularly in drug trials.

Is the exercise testing dangerous?

The purpose of testing is to stress the heart which may be diseased. Complications may occur very occasionally, so a doctor and resuscitation equipment should be immediately available. The blood pressure normally rises with exercise. If it fails to rise or, even worse, falls the test is terminated.

With these sensible precautions the risk is very small indeed. In an American study, memorable for its sheer size as well as its results, 170,000 tests were reviewed. Sixteen deaths occurred during or soon after the test (death rate 0.009 per cent). These patients often had severe heart disease; so the rate is very low. Exercise under controlled conditions with resuscitation facilities at hand is safer than uncontrolled exertion at work or leisure.

Does a normal exercise test rule out coronary artery disease?

Unfortunately, no. But it comes closer to this objective than an electrocardiogram at rest. If a patient is able to exercise up to the target heart rate without getting symptoms or electrocardiographic abnormalities, any heart disease is only mild. A common problem is the patient who is unable to exercise satisfactorily for a variety of physical of psychological reasons. Under these circumstances a negative test must be regarded as inconclusive.

Does an abnormal test always indicate coronary artery disease?

Once again, no. If the test is done with care it is fairly accurate, but it is never going to be infallible. A few false positives will always occur — tests which show electrocardiographic changes consistent with coronary artery disease when none is present. The differences between a positive and a negative test may be no more than a one millimetre shift in the tracing. The movement and rapid heart beat associated with exertion can make the tracing difficult to interpret and lead to an erroneous conclusion. Also, in a few people with normal hearts, the one millimetre shift occurs in the same manner as people with coronary heart disease. The reason for this is uncertain.

Can the exercise test determine the severity of coronary heart disease?

It is a reasonable measurement of the severity of the *symptoms* produced by the arterial disease. It is less good at assessing the number of affected vessels or the degree of narrowing. But research is being carried out to find methods of improving this.

Why is exercise testing done as a part of an athletic training programme?

This is a different use of the test; it is not done because the athletes may have heart disease. The bicycle or moving surface

29

tests are good methods for measuring the fitness of the athletes. Testing continues until the subject can do no more. Full electrocardiograms are not taken.

Ambulatory electrocardiographic monitoring (24-hour tape)

Behind this verbose term lurks a simple concept. One of the purposes of the electrocardiogram is to reveal the heart rhythm. But it will only do so for the minute or less when the recording is being made. Some of the most troublesome abnormal rhythms are those that are severe but brief in duration, perhaps only lasting a few seconds. Unless they occur very frequently the chances of catching them on a single electrocardiogram are small.

Ambulatory electrocardiographic monitoring reduces this problem by recording one or more leads of the electrocardiogram for 24 hours (24-hour tape). The technique is known as Holter monitoring in many parts of the world. At least two electrodes are stuck firmly to the chest and the signals recorded on a small portable tape recorder (Figure 3.5). The tape is driven at a slow speed so that only one cassette is needed. The patient goes about his normal activities and sleep with the recorder carried on a belt. He cannot swim or have a bath, but almost anything else is possible. The recorder will usually have an event button. This is pressed at the onset of any symptoms and enables the heart rhythm to be seen at the time when the symptoms were present.

No doctor or technician has 24 hours available to look at each 24-hour tape. So analysis has to be carried out semi-automatically. A common method is to play back the tape at 60 times normal speed. A computer can recognize most abnormal rhythms and print them out for later inspection. The operator provides an additional check by observing the rhythm on a screen as it flashes past at high speed.

Is the 24-hour tape easy to do?

For the patient the recording is a nuisance but is not particularly troublesome. The tape recorder feels much less obtrusive after it has been on for a few minutes. Sleep is easier than expected. The electrodes have to be positioned carefully and stuck on firmly. If they come off the recording will be lost.

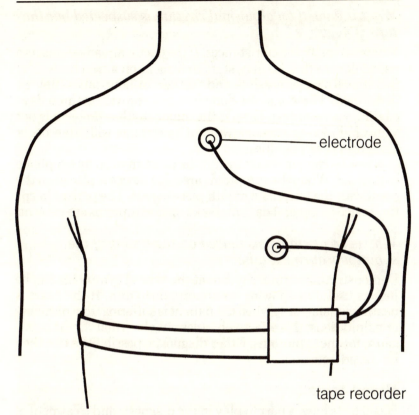

electrode

tape recorder

Figure 3.5. A 24-hour tape

How reliable is the 24-hour tape?

The 24-hour tape is the principle means of investigating rhythm problems. But the monitoring technique is entirely passive. It records events but does nothing to induce them. Any abnormal rhythms will be accurately documented if the tape is technically satisfactory. But the rhythm may not occur with sufficient frequency to be seen in a single 24-hour period. A negative 24-hour tape does not rule out an abnormal rhythm in the past, though it reduces the chances that one has occurred. So the method is very reliable if the abnormal rhythm happens during the recording, but it is much less reliable if no such rhythm takes place.

What is done if an abnormal rhythm is suspected but the tape is negative?

It depends on the circumstances. If the doctor already suspects a particular rhythm he may start treatment on a trial basis. But this is not always possible and further 24-hour tapes may be performed. Three may be done in a row, providing three days continuous recording. Even if the major rhythm problem is not 'captured', lesser versions without symptoms will often occur and give necessary clues.

A new technique is to transmit the heart rhythm by telephone to hospital. When the symptoms are felt a device is placed on the chest with the telephone mouth piece over it. The patient keeps the device for several days or weeks until symptoms are present.

Why is great emphasis placed on the timing of the symptoms during a tape?

Demonstrating normal rhythm at the time of symptoms can be just as useful as showing an abnormal rhythm. If the heart is beating satisfactorily when the patient is suffering from dizziness or palpitations, this effectively rules out abnormal rhythms as a cause for the sypmtoms. Other diagnostic possibilities can then be considered.

Blood tests

Blood tests have a part to play in the diagnosis and treatment of heart disease but they are used less than in some other medical fields. Chronic heart disease does not by itself cause blood abnormalities, but blood tests are sometimes useful in monitoring the effects on other organs and in discovering the cause of the heart damage. The use of blood tests to solve certain problems will be mentioned in later chapters.

Echocardiography

Over the last ten years echocardiography has advanced rapidly as a means of visualizing structures inside the heart. It works by the same principle that sonar (asdic) depends on to find submarines or shoals of fish. High-frequency sound waves, well above the range that can be heard by man or animals, are passed through the heart. When they hit any change in density, such as the boundary between muscle and blood, some of the waves are reflected back (Figure 3.6). With the help of suitable electronics a picture of the heart can be built up and displayed on a screen. Similar echo techniques (often referred to as ultrasound or a scan) are used to visualize the unborn baby, liver, kidneys, or other organs.

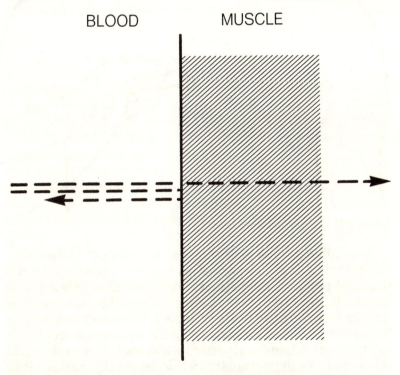

Figure 3.6. Deflection of sound waves by blood/muscle boundary

The sound waves are produced by a special crystal which is mounted in a probe and held onto the patient's chest (Figure 3.7). The waves travel easily in fluid or solid structures but are dispersed by air, so a special jelly is applied to ensure airfree contact between the probe and the chest wall. One lead of the electrocardiogram is often recorded simultaneously to time accurately contraction and relaxation of the heart.

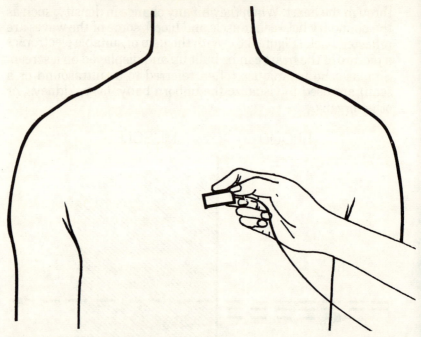

Figure 3.7. Taking an echocardiogram

Two different types of pictures can be obtained. Historically, the older is a one-dimensional picture — somewhat like the results of plunging an imaginary corkborer into the heart. The picture is displayed against time to see the movement of structures as the heart beats (M mode). The newer technique is for the beam to move from side to side like a car windscreen wiper so that a two-dimensional pattern is obtained.This method (2D echo) produces the picture that would be seen by cutting a thin slice from the heart. It is displayed on a television screen to show the movement of structures. With both techniques the beam is pointed in various directions to build up a more complete impression of the heart. The two methods provide different information and are complementary to each other.

Does echocardiography hurt?

No. The sound waves produce no sensation at all and are too high pitched to be heard. They are quite harmless.

What is echocardiography used for?

Echocardiography is particularly good at revealing the shape and movement of structures within the heart. They cannot be seen on the ordinary chest X-ray. For example, the mitral valve cannot be detected on the chest X-ray but its structure can be seen in detail with the echocardiogram. The information that echocardiography provides could often be got by cardiac catheterization, but echocardiography is much more convenient. It can also repeated many times if necessary, enabling the progress of the disease to be followed.

Can echocardiography be used in children?

Heart disease in children is largely a problem of incorrect development of the heart. Echocardiography is very suitable for seeing the disordered valves and cardiac chambers that are produced. As nothing is felt it can be readily done in children. It is especially useful in the new-born who are difficult to investigate by other means. Nowadays cardiac structures can be seen by echocardiography while the baby is still inside the womb.

Will echocardiography work in everybody?

Most people, but not everybody. The sound waves travel in straight lines in fluid or solid structures but are dispersed by air. So the beam will be scattered by traversing air in the lungs. Fortunately the lungs do not cover the front of the heart in most people and the beam can be directed to the correct place. The operator may ask the subject to lie on his left side to move the lungs out of the way. But a few people, particularly smokers with expanded lungs, do not have this gap and echocardiography is difficult or impossible. A deformed chest wall can be a problem as the beam has to be directed between the ribs.

Can it be wrong?

Like all investigations, echocardiography depends on correct interpretation and this can occasionally be wrong. Good judgement is required both by the person who is doing the echocardiography and by the doctor who reviews the pictures. Experience is essential. Overall, echocardiograms are reliable as long as the conclusions are cautious and fully justified by the pictures.

If the echocardiogram is so good, why are other investigations done?

In many patients no further investigations are needed, but in others it does not provide all the answers. Echocardiography looks at structures, so it will not measure pressures inside the heart which are often essential to determine the severity of a lesion. It will not help with rhythm problems, except to suggest an underlying cause. Also the sound beam is not sufficiently fine to see small structures. A common problem is that coronary arteries are not visible with current echocardiographic techniques and cardiac catheterization is required to see them.

Isotope scanning

Isotope scanning of the heart is a new test whose importance is not yet fully assessed. A small quantity of a mildly radioactive chemical is injected into the circulation through a vein. Some of the radioactivity will be taken up by the heart. By using a device somewhat like a sophisticated geiger counter a picture of the radioactivity defining the heart muscle is obtained.

As the technique is new, different methods are still being explored. A common one is to inject radioactive thallium. If the blood flow to the heart muscle is obstructed by coronary artery narrowing or blockage, the affected muscle will be underperfused by the thallium-containing blood. The resulting radioactive defect can be detected by the scanner and used to estimate the degree of coronary artery narrowing. This method can be made more accurate by observing the changes that take place with exercise. The underlying concept is attractive as in theory the radioactivity is providing a direct measurement of blood flow to the heart muscle.

Another method is to scan the radioactive material (for example technetium) as it passes through the left ventricular cavity. This outlines the movement of the ventricular wall and is a guide to the state of health of the ventricular muscle. The resulting picture is similar, but not as accurate as the left ventricular angiogram done at catheterization.

These methods are quite safe as the amount of radioactivity is minimal — less than many X-ray procedures. At present the technique can provide useful information, but it is not sufficiently reliable. Only large structures can be seen. So far, isotope scanning is a supporting investigation; not the test that will provide the answer by itself. However, this may change in the course of future development.

Cardiac catheterization

Cardiac catheterization (the passage of a tube into the heart) is one of the foundation stones of modern cardiology. The development of heart surgery and our understanding of how the human heart works are derived from it. In 1929 Forssmann was the first person to catheterize the human heart — his own! The technique was thought to be highly dangerous and was not accepted as a useful test. Forssmann went off to an undistinguished career as a kidney and bladder sugeon. Times changed and he was brought back in 1956 to receive jointly a Nobel prize. Today cardiac catheterization is a common test, especially in the assessment of possible heart surgery. It requires expertise and expensive equipment so the majority of catherizations are performed in cardiac investigation centres.

To gain entry into the heart the tube (catheter) is passed into a large artery or vein and then moved towards the heart. The position of the catheter is followed on an X-ray screen. If the catheter is inserted into a vein it will go into the right atrium, then through into the right ventricle and the artery to the lungs (right heart catheterization: Figure 3.8). If it is placed in the artery it will be pushed backwards up the artery into the left ventricle (left heart catheterization). Alternatively, to enter the left atrium and ventricle, a catheter can be passed up a vein into the right atrium and then pushed through the thin wall of atrial muscle into the left atrium. Right and left heart catheterizations are often done simultaneously.

The pressure inside the heart can be measured. The catheter is filled with water so the pressure at the tip is transmitted down the tube. The end outside the body is connected to a pressure-measuring device (transducer) which displays the changing pressure as a line on a piece of paper. The pressure at any point of the cardiac cycle of contraction can be found by inspecting this tracing. The catheter is moved to different parts of the heart and the pressures recorded in turn. A large amount of information about the degree of heart damage or the narrowness of the valves can be derived from these measurements. Sometimes the

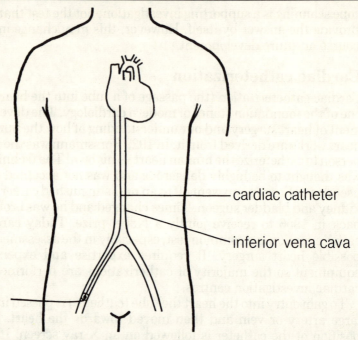

cardiac catheter

inferior vena cava

Figure 3.8. Right heart catheterization from the groin

patient is asked to exercise his arms or legs while lying on the catheterization table. Exercise tends to magnify any pressure abnormalities.

Catheterization can be used to detect and locate abnormal holes within the heart. Blood samples are taken by pulling back with a syringe on the end of the catheter. The oxygen contents of these samples from different sites are measured. In the normal heart the oxygen content in the blood from the right atrium, right ventricle, and the artery to the lungs are all low, but similar. If a hole in the heart is present, blood with a high content of oxygen may travel from the left atrium or ventricle into the right side of the heart. The resulting change in oxygen concentration can be detected by sampling at different sites in the right heart.

Cardiac catheterization is often used to display structures which are inside, or just outside, the heart. A special solution that shows up on X-ray (contrast medium) is pumped into a cardiac chamber through the catheter. The chamber is briefly filled with the contrast medium and the solid structures of the heart muscle and valves appear as shadows within or around the medium. The medium leaking backwards through a faulty valve can also be seen. The pictures are recorded on film or video for later detailed inspection. The technique is known as angiography. A special type of angiography is coronary arteriography. The two coronary arteries supply blood to the heart muscle itself. After inserting a catheter into a coronary artery, contrast medium is injected down to reveal any narrowed or blocked portions. Coronary arteriography is essential when surgery on these arteries is being considered. In Europe and North America the need to perform coronary arteriography is now the commonest reason for cardiac catheterization.

What happens at a cardiac catheterization?

Different methods are used, even within one hospital. The principles are the same but the details vary. The following description is a guide but will not be correct in every case.

A brief admission to hospital is usually, but not always, required. Shortly before the procedure the patient is mildly sedated with tablets or an injection to make him relaxed. Food and drink is withheld for a few hours beforehand, as vomiting might spoil the results or make any complications more troublesome. On arrival at the catheterization room the patient is confronted by nurses, technicians and doctors, all wearing masks and special clothing. It will probably remind him of operating theatres seen in television drama series. This is no accident; the degree of sterility required in a catheterization room is the same as that needed in an operating theatre. Many of the staff will be wearing leadlined jackets. The room seems to be full of equipment. The X-ray apparatus and cine camera are moved close to the table. The X-ray controls are behind a screen. Elsewhere in the room will be the pressure-recording devices, a screen to see the pictures, a trolley with instruments, and a pump to deliver the contrast medium for angiography.

The catheters are inserted into the arm or the groin. After cleaning the skin and arranging the sterile towels, local anaesthetic is injected. If the arm is being used, a small cut is made. Then the artery and vein are dissected out and the catheters inserted into them. With the groin route the catheters are manoeuvred straight into the vessels; no dissection is required. For this method, a needle is first inserted into the artery or vein. A fine wire is passed into the vessel through the needle. The needle is removed, leaving the wire in place. The catheter is then advanced down the wire and into the vessel. The wire is finally taken out, leaving the catheter in the artery or vein.

The doctor moves the catheters to the appropriate part of the heart. In some patients this is easy, but in others it can take longer. The catheters have special shapes to enable them to go into particular places — for example, the coronary arteries. Sometimes the catheter is taken out and replaced by a different-shaped one during the procedure. The doctor may ask the patient to exercise his arms or legs so that the heart is stressed and abnormalities magnified. Most catheterizations include some angiography. The best pictures are taken with an X-ray beam at an angle to the chest. To get the correct angle the X-ray beam is tilted to one side. Alternatively the beam stays fixed and the patient is rotated, using a special cradle and straps to hold him firmly in place.

The duration of a catheterization depends on the number of pressure measurements, oxygen saturations, and X-ray pictures that are required. It normally lasts from 30 minutes to 2 hours. At the end the catheters are removed. An artery in the arm will be closed with a small suture. A vein in the arm is just tied off as the blood will flow through one of many alternative veins. In the groin the artery and vein are sealed by pressing on them for several minutes. An arm wound will be closed with a couple of stitches. The needle pricks in the leg are much smaller and no stitches are needed.

Does cardiac catheterization hurt?

This varies from test to test. Some patients claim afterwards to have felt hardly anything at all, while others have noticed rather more. Some slight discomfort is inevitable but it is nearly always much less than the patient anticipates. The needle prick of the local anaesthetic cannot be avoided and the anaesthetic agent itself often produces a stinging feeling as it stimulates the small nerves before blocking them. During most catheterizations at least one hot flush will be felt from the contrast medium. For angiography the medium is injected into the middle of the heart. The medium is denser than blood and produces a hot feeling for the few seconds that the heart takes to pump it around the body.

The doctor will normally warn the patient that the medium is about to be injected.

These sensations are part of most catheterizations but they are often the only discomfort. Patients are always surprised to find that the movement of the catheter inside the body produces little or no sensation. The inside of blood vessels has no nerves to register that movement. If such nerves existed we would be kept awake all night by the movement of the blood. Rarely, the catheter catches and tugs on a vessel branch to produce brief discomfort. Pain can be produced by an artery which is too small for the catheter, which is then changed to a smaller size. Angina sufferers may find that the pain is brought on by the catheterization. The catheters may induce extra beats as they enter the heart. The beats can sometimes be felt but are not painful. In general, the procedure is not particularly distressing, no worse than a visit to the dentist. Older patients tend to doze off during warm afternoon sessions.

Is cardiac catheterization dangerous?

Cardiac catheterization is the equivalent of a minor operation. It carries a small, but definite, risk. The chance of an important complication is very small and difficult to quantify. Many of the patients have severe heart disease and any deterioration is not necessarily due to the catheterization. Many doctors have had the experience of postponing a test for technical reasons and then finding that the patient has become more ill on the day when the test would have taken place. If the catheterization had gone ahead the deterioration would have been attributed to it. The risk will vary with the severity of the underlying heart disease. If a patient is already deteriorating rapidly the dangers are much greater. Leaving aside these high-risk unstable patients, a dangerous complication could be expected to occur once in every 250-500 tests in an average heart unit. By prompt action many of these dangers can be controlled.

Many of the complications of catheterization are minor troubles related to the closure of the artery. Persistent bleeding is an example. The catheter may disturb the heart rhythm, but this is usually either unimportant or can be corrected immediately. Perforation of the heart is a rare, but serious problem; an emergency operation to close the hole is then required. The accidental introduction of air or blood clot into the circulation is another rare complication. It can be dangerous if the air or clot travels in the blood stream and lodges in an artery elsewhere in the body. The obstruction of the artery may damage the organ it supplies. Rarely, coronary arteriography precipitates a heart attack. If the coronary artery is already severely narrowed, the insertion of a catheter and the injection of contrast medium may be the final straw.

Although these serious complications are uncommon, they do occur and in a particular patient they can be a major problem. So catheterization is only done if the necessary information cannot be obtained by other means. On the other hand, catheterization is performed to find the correct treatment of heart disease, a potentially dangerous condition. The risk of not doing the test, and providing the wrong treatment, are much greater than the risks of doing it.

When is catheterization performed?

Possible cardiac surgery is the commonest indication. The advantages and hazards of surgery can only be assessed if the nature and severity of the disease is clearly defined. Echocardiography can sometimes provide the necessary information but catheterization is needed on most occasions.

At times catheterization is performed for monitoring drug therapy. One example is the treatment of heart failure in the coronary care unit soon after a heart attack. A special catheter is introduced into a vein and floated through the heart. Its position is determined by the pressure measurements; no X-rays are used. Occasionally catheterization is performed for reasons related to the patient's job. A typical example is an airline pilot with chest pains that could be coming from his heart. Unless his coronary arteries can be shown to be normal by angiography, he will lose his job.

Are there any after-effects?

Slight bruising around the site where the catheter entered the artery is common. Sometimes it is more than slight. As a precaution against bleeding the patients are rested afterwards. Any bleeding is controlled by firm pressure. The mild sedation that is given beforehand tends to induce sleepiness once the excitement is over. In general patients are back to normal within a few hours. From the day after the test patients can return to their previous level of activity.

Why do the staff wear lead-lined jackets in the catheterization room?

Only a minimal amount of radiation is produced by the X-rays from one catheterization. But the staff, who may be participating in several hundreds of tests per year, are exposed to much more than one patient. The lead-lined jackets are a shield over their bodies to minimize the amount of radiation received.

Can children be catheterized?

Yes. Newborn babies are often catheterized in centres dealing with heart disease in the very young. Children find lying still difficult and can be frightened by the injection of local anaesthetic. So the test is often performed under general anaesthesia or heavy sedation in young children.

Electrophysiology

Electrophysiology testing is a method of exploring the passage of electrical signals through the heart. These signals should maintain the normal rhythm of the heart. A good impression of these internal signals can be obtained from the standard external electrocardiogram, but more detailed information is available with electrophysiological studies. Special catheter electrodes are used. They are not tubes like ordinary catheters, but solid structures with wires inside leading to a number of electrodes at the end. The electrodes are positioned within the heart to record the spread of electricity. The techniques for inserting the catheter electrodes are the same as those used for ordinary catheters. But more catheter electrodes are employed — up to five in some patients.

Electrophysiology is fairly new and its place in the investigation of heart disease is still small. Its main use is in disentangling complex rhythm problems, particularly those resistant to drug treatment. Under these circumstances it is very helpful, but most rhythm problems can be managed without it.

Conclusion

The range and power of modern cardiac investigations can resolve almost any problem. This is potentially both a boon and a curse to the patient. A boon because genuine uncertainties can be speedily resolved if required. A curse because the patient can be over-investigated when the precise diagnosis is already clear, or is irrelevant to the treatment. The latter course is more common in litigation-prone North America than in Britain, where financial constraints limit the number of tests. Fortunately an account of the symptoms and an examination, supplemented if necessary by a simple chest X-ray or electrocardiogram, will solve most problems in suspected heart disease. But it is comforting to know that the complex tests are there if needed.

4

Angina and heart attacks

Angina and heart attacks are produced by an insufficient blood flow to the heart muscle. This is normally, but not always, due to disease of the coronary arteries. Atherosclerosis is by far the commonest cause and so represents the most important agent of heart disease in the developed world. A deficiency in the blood supply to an organ is known as ischaemia so this coronary artery disease is also called ischaemic heart disease. It can display itself in a number of ways.

The four major subdivisions are angina, myocardial infarction, intermediate syndrome, and sudden cardiac death. A patient may have more than one of these manifestations of ischaemic heart disease; an unlucky patient could develop all four.

Angina

Strictly speaking, the correct term is 'angina pectoris'. 'Angina' is an old medical word for a spasmodic pain. For example, Vincent's angina is a type of painful mouth infection. 'Pectoris' means that the spasmodic pain is felt in the chest. Nowadays the second word is usually missed out and 'angina' by itself always means a spasmodic pain in the chest secondary to insufficient blood flow in the coronary arteries.

Myocardial infarction

Infarction is destruction of cells due to an inadequate blood supply. So myocardial infarction means that some of the heart muscle (myocardium) is permanently damaged by ischaemia. Heart attack is an imprecise term, but when doctors use it they mean a myocardial infarction.

Intermediate syndrome

This cumbersome term refers to something between angina and a myocardial infarction. The chest pain is too persistent or frequent for angina but the heart muscle has not been damaged. Other terms are used to describe particular forms of this intermediate syndrome, such as unstable angina or acute coronary insufficiency.

Sudden cardiac death

A few unfortunate people suddenly become ill with heart disease and die within minutes. Until recently it was assumed that this sudden cardiac death was the result of a severe myocardial infarction. Sometimes it is, but we now know that it is possible to die suddenly from heart disease without an infarction. This problem is important and to avoid prejudging the cause of death it is best to regard sudden cardiac death as a distinct manifestation of ischaemic heart disease.

Atherosclerosis

What is atherosclerosis?

Atherosclerosis, also know as atheroma, is the deposition of fats and other substances in the wall of an artery, narrowing its lumen (Figure 4.1). The eventual result may be complete blockage of the artery. In addition the atherosclerosis produces a rough vessel wall which is a potential site for a blood clot. Partial obstruction by atherosclerosis can be made worse by local clotting (thrombosis).

Which vessels develop atherosclerosis?

Any artery in the body can be affected. Veins are immune. In this book we are largely concerned with the coronary arteries. Atherosclerosis is characteristically a patchy disease. One artery can be severely affected while another is normal. A vessel can be narrowed in one place but be unaffected elsewhere.

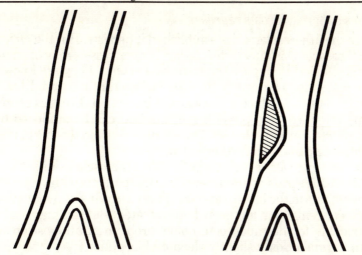

Figure 4.1 Left — a normal blood vessel. Right — atherosclerosis narrowing the blood vessel

What causes atherosclerosis?

If we knew the full answer to this question we could probably prevent coronary artery disease. Some people are vulnerable to developing atherosclerosis while the others are resistant. Certain factors are associated with its occurrence. Preventable ones include cigarette smoking, high blood pressure, and a high level of some blood fats. Others such as increasing age, being male, and a familial incidence of atherosclerosis cannot be altered. The topic will be discussed later in this chapter and in chapter eight.

These factors predispose people to coronary artery disease but they are not the only causes of it. A few unfortunate women develop atherosclerosis in spite of having none of these factors. Conversely, some men have all of them but avoid arterial disease. Other unknown influences are at work.

At what age does atherosclerosis start?

Mild atherosclerosis can sometimes be seen in the coronary arteries of teenage boys but it rarely produces any significant disease until after 30 years of age. A few children with very high levels of blood fats or other rare diseases may develop coronary artery disease but this is very unusual.

Does atherosclerosis regress?

Once the atherosclerosis is established it persists. But the *effects* of atherosclerosis may be temporary. Other vessels may open up to allow blood to bypass the narrowed artery. They are known as collaterals. The artery may be sufficiently narrowed for a thrombosis to produce a myocardial infarction. But this represents the maximum possible damage that can be produced by this patch of atherosclerosis. Once it has occurred this particular narrowing can do no further harm.

It is a controversial point whether the atherosclerosis itself can be made to regress by treatment. In a few patients with very high levels of fats in the blood, reversal of the narrowing by a reduction in fat concentration has been demonstrated. But this may not be applicable to the much commoner problem of atherosclerosis with normal or only slightly elevated blood fats.

Can atherosclerosis be detected before it produces heart disease?

Atherosclerosis can be present for decades before any heart disease is apparent. Unfortunately we have no easy and reliable method of detecting early arterial disease in patients without overt heart trouble.

The electrocardiogram has been suggested as a possible means of screening for atherosclerosis. It can be abnormal, particularly during exercise (p.26), before any symptoms occur. But the changes in the tracing are not very specific and atherosclerosis may be diagnosed incorrectly. Conversely, the electrocardiogram can be normal when a significant degree of coronary artery disease is present. The electrocardiogram is not a good screening test though it is sometimes used in people such as airline pilots when the consequences of sudden heart disease might be disastrous.

Angina

What is angina?

Angina is a type of heart pain. The nature of this pain, which is often 'crushing' and in the middle of the chest, has been described in Chapter 3. The key element in the diagnosis of angina is that the pain comes on during exercise or emotion and is relieved by a few minutes rest. Walking up a hill or carrying shopping home are typical methods of inducing it. Cold weather or a heavy meal also increase the demands on the heart so exercise under these circumstances is particularly liable to produce the pain. It should be emphasized that the discomfort comes on *during* exertion or emotion. Pain that starts once exercise is finished is unlikely to be angina.

What causes angina?

This was also discussed in Chapter 3. The commonest cause is atherosclerotic coronary artery narrowing producing an insufficient blood flow for the greatly increased needs of the heart muscles during exercise (Figure 4.2). The heart can manage satisfactorily at rest, but with exercise insufficient oxygen is reaching the cells. Another possible cause is normal coronary arteries being unable to supply enough blood to an abnormally thick heart muscle. Thick muscle often needs more oxygen, particularly during exercise. The thickening is often in response to an obstruction in the outflow from the left ventricle such as narrowing of the aortic valve (aortic stenosis).

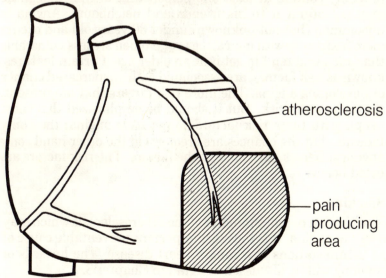

atherosclerosis

pain producing area

Figure 4.2. Atherosclerosis in a coronary artery producing angina

Is the heart damaged by angina?

Angina is an effective 'safety valve', preventing damage to the heart. When the shortage of oxygen produces the pain of angina no permanent injury has occurred. The pain stops further exercise, allowing the heart to recover quickly. So a patient with angina can exercise until he gets the pain without any worry that the heart will be damaged. But he should stop and rest as soon as the discomfort starts. Once it has gone exercise can continue.

A few people with angina notice that if they force themselves to carry on during an attack, the pain disappears in a few minutes and does not return ('walk-through angina'). This may be dangerous; it is similar to tying down the safety valve of a steam engine. Angina is a form of heart protection and should not be ignored.

Who gets angina?

Angina is a common problem. So common that it is impossible to know how many people have it. An average bus-load will probably contain at least one person with angina though he may not admit it to his friends and neighbours. Angina is uncommon (but not unknown) under 30 years old and occurs more frequently with increasing age. Women are less vulnerable than men and tend to get it at an older age. Certain features, known as risk factors, are associated with an increased chance of developing angina. The more risk factors that are present, the greater the risk. But it should be emphasized that most people with these risk factors do not have angina; they only indicate that the chances are greater. On the other hand some angina sufferers have none of the factors. The risk factors are listed below.

Smoking

Smoking is a potent promoter of the atherosclerosis which may result in angina. It is the most important preventable cause of all manifestations of coronary heart disease. The hazards of smoking will be discussed in detail in Chapter 8.

Hypertension

High blood pressure (hypertension) is associated with an increased incidence of angina. The increased pressure in the coronary arteries encourages the formation of atherosclerosis. In addition the heart has to work harder to pump the blood at a pressure higher than normal. This requires more oxygen which increases the significance of any coronary artery narrowing.

Increased blood fats

The fats in the blood are referred to as lipids; excess fats in the blood is called hyperlipidaemia. It is a controversial subject which has generated much research in the last thirty years. The best known and easiest to measure lipid is cholesterol. Triglyceride is another type. No doubt exists that an increased concentration of cholesterol and triglyceride is associated with a greater risk of angina and other forms of coronary artery disease. But a fierce controversy still rages as to how much the risk is diminished by a reduction in the lipid concentrations by diet or drugs. Let us leave this interesting topic to Chapter 8.

Diabetes

Patients with diabetes are also more vulnerable to angina. Their arteries show an increased incidence of atherosclerosis though only a minority of diabetics develop the disease.

Underactive thyroid gland

A long-standing deficiency of thyroxine, the thyroid gland hormone, can produce atherosclerosis and angina. This is uncommon nowadays as an underactive thyroid gland (hypothyroidism) can be easily treated.

Lack of exercise

The absence of frequent exercise is associated with an increased chance of developing angina though we are still uncertain how important this is. It is another important topic for Chapter 8.

Familial incidence

Angina is not an inherited disease; it is not passed down from parents to children. Nevertheless members of some families seem to have higher chance of developing it than those in other families.

This factor should not be overemphasized as the increased risk is not great. Its main importance is in identifying families whose members should pay particular attention to the prevention of coronary artery disease.

Obesity

The importance of obesity by itself as a significant risk factor is undecided. Excess weight is certainly associated with an increased incidence of angina, but the obesity is often combined with other risk factors such as hypertension, lack of exercise, increased blood fats, and diabetes. It may be that these other factors are the ones producing the greater risk of angina. But whatever the mechanism, weight reduction has a part to play in the control of angina.

Does stress cause angina?

This common question is difficult to answer. The belief that stress is a factor in the genesis of coronary artery disease is persistent, but it is not backed by good evidence. But proof would be hard to obtain. Stress is very difficult to measure making it an unsuitable subject for accurate scientific study. An acute stress may precipitate an attack of angina by forcing the heart to beat faster and work harder. Whether chronic stress is involved in the formation of atherosclerosis, the underlying problem in angina, is uncertain. The increased risk of angina in developed countries is sometimes cited as evidence that stress is important. But the assumption that life in a westernized city is more 'stressful' than eking out a basic existence under extreme poverty is dubious and a little arrogant. This topic will be mentioned again in Chapter 8.

Why do people without risk factors get angina?

These factors point to men and women with an increased risk of developing angina. But some angina sufferers do not have any. It used to be thought that everybody would get coronary artery disease if they lived long enough. The idea was that some individuals developed it earlier than others. But we now realize that coronary arteries can remain normal in spite of advancing years. Additional, unknown, factors help to promote atherosclerosis and the resulting angina. It is a pity that we cannot yet identify them.

What tests are required?

No tests are required to diagnose a straightforward example of angina. The patient's story will suffice. Nothing may be found on examination. In a more difficult case the electrocardiogram can be very helpful. A normal electrocardiogram does not exclude angina, but abnormalities in the tracings can support a suspected diagnosis. An exercise electrocardiogram (p.26) can be even more useful, but the best way to diagnose angina is to talk to the patient. An electrocardiogram taken in isolation can be very misleading.

Does angina ever disappear spontaneously?

Yes, more often than people realize. A quarter of patients who develop angina find that it disappears within a few months. In others it is only an intermittent problem, perhaps confined to cold winter days. Treatment will increase the number of patients who are no longer troubled by angina.

Are patients with angina liable to have a heart attack?

Unfortunately anybody may develop a myocardial infarction at some time. In some of us the risk is low, but doctors can never say that a particular person has no chance of ever suffering an infarction.

Angina and a myocardial infarction are produced by different mechanisms though they do share the same origin — coronary artery disease. Most patients with stable angina do not go on to have an infarction, particularly if risk factors are modified as necessary. But it is still true that the chance of an infarction is increased in comparison to subjects without angina. The risk is small but it indicates that angina should always be considered seriously and treated appropriately.

What is crescendo angina?

This description means that the angina is worsening rapidly. For example, the distance walked before the onset of pain get progressively shorter over a few days until the patient can hardly move across a room. The risk of developing an infarction during crescendo angina is greater than during stable angina. Immediate therapy is required, usually bed rest and drugs. The majority of cases settle with treatment and no infarction occurs. Occasionally the crescendo angina does not resolve and coronary artery vein grafting may be the best way of solving the problem (p.160).

Can the pain of angina be distinguished from the pain of a myocardial infarction?

Both conditions produce the same cardiac pain. An important property of the pain in angina is that it is relieved by a few minutes rest, while the discomfort of an infarction persists longer. So a heart pain which lasts for less than ten minutes is not produced by an infarction. It may still not be an infarction when the pain lasts longer but urgent medical advice should be sought if the persisting discomfort is a new phenomenon.

What can relieve an attack of angina?

The person must stop exercising or, if the attack is secondary to emotion, calm down. The discomfort will go within minutes. 'Burping' sometimes relieves the pain; the heart and the gullet (oesophagus) share a common nerve supply and release of any stomach distention seems to help.

Drugs can be used to shorten an attack. Placing a nitrate tablet under the tongue and allowing it to dissolve works in most people. If the tablets are swallowed the nitrates will not be absorbed fast enough to abort an attack. Two common nitrates are glyceryl trinitrate and isosorbide dinitrate. Some preparations are designed to be chewed rather than left to dissolve under the tongue. The main unwanted effect of all nitrate tablets is a throbbing headache which some patients feel is worse than the chest pain. This can be minimized by spitting out the tablet as soon as the angina is relieved. A reduced dose may also help. In a few people the nitrates drop the blood pressure and produce transient dizziness, which can be alarming on the first occasion but it is not dangerous.

What can prevent an attack of angina?

The chronic treatment of angina requires a combined approach by the patient and his doctor. The aim is to abolish the attacks or at least to increase the amount of exercise that can be tolerated.

The patient has to lose excess weight. Walking with an extra 10 kilograms of body fat is like carrying a suitcase of the same weight; the pain will start sooner. Smoking will have to be abandoned. A period of rest may be required if the angina has just appeared or is getting worse, but exercise should not be limited unnecessarily. The old view was that angina sufferers should always 'take it easy'. But it has now been shown that patients with *stable* angina and no other medical problem do better if they exercise regularly. Exertion encourages the heart to work more efficiently. It is quite safe as long as it is stopped as soon as the pain occurs.

In addition to giving advice the doctor will often prescribe drugs to control angina. The tablets or capsules are taken one to three times a day indefinitely. They are designed to prevent attacks, not to relieve them, so they have to be taken every day. Not suprisingly the pharmaceutical industry has brought out a large number of drugs to fill this lucrative market. The main classes of drugs are listed below.

Beta blockers

Common examples: propranolol (Inderal), oxprenolol (Trasicor), atenolol (Trenormin), metroprolol (Lopressor, Betaloc).

Advantages: effective and well tolerated in most patients, also useful in hypertension, abnormal heart rhythms, and other conditions

Disadvantages: can worsen asthma, heart failure, or poor circulation to the legs.

Side-effects: cold extremities, nightmares, tiredness.

Long-acting nitrates

Common examples: isosorbide dinitrate, slow-release nitrate preparations, nitrate ointments (large number of different trade names.

Advantages: good for heart failure.

Disadvantages: variable effectiveness, have to be taken several times a day.

Side-effects: headaches can be a problem though less than with nitrates being used to relieve an attack.

Calcium antagonists

Common examples: nifedipine (Adalat), verapamil (Cordilox).
Advantages: few side-effects, combine well with beta blockers,
   also useful in hypertension.
Disadvantages: probably less effective but trials still going on.
Side-effects: rare.

The response of a patient to these drugs cannot be predicted in
advance. So several may need to be tried in turn at differing doses
before the most effective treatment is found. All drugs can
produce side-effects in a few people, but these are usually well
tolerated. Some problems, such as the headache produced by a
nitrate preparation, are temporary and rarely persist after the
first few days. A doctor may recommend that the patient should
carry on with the drug rather than stop it prematurely because of
transient side-effects.

The distinction between prevention of angina and relief of an
attack is useful in practice but should not be too rigid. For
example, nifedipine is a calcium antagonist formulated for
swallowing three times a day to prevent angina. But the same
capsule will often relieve an attack if it is chewed in the mouth.
Alternatively, if an angina sufferer knows that a walk up a hill
may bring on the pain, he can place a glyceryl trinitrate tablet
under his tongue before he starts and get up the hill without
difficulty.

Can surgery help angina?

One of the major advances in the treatment of heart disease in the
last few years is the ability to control angina by surgery. The
diseased areas of the coronary arteries are identified precisely by
cardiac catheterization and coronary arteriography (p.39) and
vein grafts are used to bypass the narrowings. By this means
unimpeded blood flow is restored to the heart muscle. The
operation, known as coronary artery vein grafting, will be
described in more detail in Chapter 7.

Which patients with angina will benefit from an operation?

Coronary artery vein grafting is done for two reasons. The commoner one is to control angina which has not responded to drug

treatment, weight loss, and cessation of smoking. The other indication is to prevent a myocardial infarction in the future by relieving critical obstructions in the coronary arteries.

The operation is very effective in treating intractable angina. About three patients out of four have total relief of their pain and do not require further drug therapy. In the remainder the angina is usually considerably improved though they may need to continue on long-term treatment. The operation is worth contemplating in most young or middle aged patients whose angina is interfering with their life despite drug therapy. What constitute interference will depend on the person and his activities. A manual worker will be less able to tolerate the pain than an office worker. The operation should be considered in anybody who is thinking about an unwanted change of jobs or premature retirement because angina is upsetting his work.

But many such patients will not have surgery. The patient may prefer to accept limitations on his activities rather than go through the discomfort and small risk of surgery. Other illnesses might mean that the operation would carry an unacceptably high degree of risk. An inability to lose weight or give up smoking may make the doctors unenthusiastic for such a costly, involved, procedure. The coronary artery disease may be widespread; so no normal artery remains for the attachment of the vein grafts. Under these circumstances the results of surgery will probably be worse than the results of drug therapy so an operation is not advisable. Sometimes the heart has already been significantly damaged by previous infarctions. This reduces the chances of a good surgical result.

The other indication for vein grafting is to prevent trouble in the future. Heart specialists have different opinions about this controversial subject. A major difficulty is that coronary artery disease can be an evolving process. In some patients the damaged areas of the arteries may remain unchanged for years, but in others fresh obstructions appear in previously unaffected arteries. It can be difficult to predict whether a particular patient will benefit from the protective effects of surgery.

For the majority of patients vein grafting is a good method of relieving angina, but it does not seem to alter the risk of an infarction in the future. However, this is not true for all patients. For example, about one in ten of those being considered for operation have an obstruction in the left main artery before it divides into the two branches (p.9). This narrowing will effect the blood supply to a large area of the heart so there is a significant chance of a large infarction at some time. The extra risk is reduced by vein grafting; for this sub-group surgery will diminish the chance of future trouble. The operation may also reduce the risk of infarction if all three major coronary arteries are narrowed; not all experts agree on this. Research is continuing and other sub-groups who will benefit may be identified soon.

Atypical angina

Angina normally comes on with exercise or emotion, and is relieved by rest. But in a few patients the angina is not produced by these means; this is known as atypical angina. The pain is the same as ordinary angina, but the circumstances when it occurs are atypical. Variant angina is another name.

What causes atypical angina

Spasm of the coronary arteries is the precipitating factor. The blood flow is usually already reduced by some fixed athersoscler-otic narrowings. The additional diminution in blood to the heart muscle creates an oxygen shortage, producing the pain. The spasm only lasts for a few minutes; blood then flows back to the muscle and the pain goes. As yet we do not know what causes the spasm. It can occur at any time.

How is atypical angina diagnosed?

It can be very difficult. The problem is to distinguish atypical angina from other pains which are not coming from the heart. Non-cardiac pain is common while atypical angina is rare. Transitory electrocardiographic changes occur during atypical angina and are the best means of establishing the diagnosis. In hospital an electrocardiogram can be taken during the pain. Outside hospital ambulatory monitoring (p.30) can sometimes be used to document the changes.

How is it treated?

Drugs which reverse the coronary artery spasm are the most useful. Nitrate tablets allowed to dissolve under the tongue may help as they do in more typical forms of angina. Long-acting drugs such as certain nitrate preparations and calcium antagonists (verapamil, nifedipine) may prevent both types of angina. In theory beta blockers are helpful in ordinary angina but may worsen atypical angina by promoting spasm. However, we do not know how important this effect is in practice.

Myocardial infarction

What is myocardial infarction?

A myocardial infarction is permanent damage to some of the heart muscle cells produced by a prolonged period of insufficient blood supply and resulting oxygen deprivation. The cells lose all contractile function and do not recover. Over the following 4-6 weeks they are replaced by fibrous tissue which creates the equivalent of a scar.

What is a heart attack?

Unfortunately this term has different meanings. One meaning is synonymous with a myocardial infarction. At times it is widened to include the intermediate syndrome or sudden cardiac death. It may be used to refer to any sudden event affecting the heart. Non-medical people may stretch its meaning even further to encompass sudden events involving the blood vessels as well, for example a stroke. Because of this ambiguity the term 'heart attack' is not often used in this book.

An older description of a myocardial infarction is coronary thrombosis. The term refers to the commonest cause of myocardial infarction, a thrombosis, or clot, in a coronary artery. But not every infarction is secondary to such a thrombosis and the thrombosis does not always produce an infarction. So the older term is used less often today in medical circles. People often talk about somebody having a 'coronary'. Strictly speaking this does not make sense as the word is just an adjective that can be applied to anything related to the coronary arteries. But by common usage it is taken to mean a coronary thrombosis.

What causes a myocardial infarction?

Like angina the underlying problem is disease of the coronary arteries, usually atherosclerosis. But the immediate events are different. For many years doubt existed as to whether the cause of infarction was progression of the atherosclerotic narrowing of the coronary artery or whether it was a thrombus forming inside a diseased vessel. Recent work indicates that most infarctions are due to thrombus formation in a narrowed, but not blocked, coronary artery (Figure 4.3). Angina is produced by a fairly constant blood flow being unable to keep up with the increased demands of the heart muscle. In contrast, for a myocardial infarction the demands of the muscles are constant but the blood flow is markedly reduced.

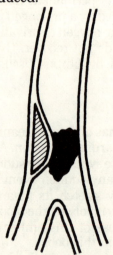

Figure 4.3. Formation of an infarction

In practical terms this means that an infarction is not produced by exercise or emotion. If it is going to occur it can start at any time. Unlike angina, exercise is not the precipitating factor, so the pain is not relieved by rest. The discomfort persists until it is terminated by treatment or the cells are permanently damaged. Once the area of the heart muscle is non-functional the effects of the oxygen shortage are no longer felt and the pain goes.

What produces the coronary artery thrombosis?
We do not yet have a complete answer to this problem. We do

know that thrombosis only occurs in arteries which are already diseased. An infarction is extremely rare with normal coronary arteries, though it can occur. Under these circumstances other forms of heart disease are responsible. In general the risk of thrombosis is related to the severity of the coronary artery disease. But the relationship is not always accurate. Some severely diseased vessels never seem to develop thrombosis while an infarction can occur secondary to a thrombus in an artery with only moderate narrowing.

The formation of the thrombus is imperfectly understood. If an artery is cut, thrombus formation is a natural method of staunching the bleeding. Thrombi do not occur in an intact, healthy, artery. But a diseased artery can have the same effect on the blood as a cut artery; the internal lining is no longer intact and a thrombus is created. We do not know why this clotting affects some diseased arteries but not others. The viscosity (thickness) of the blood may be important. The fats in the blood may also be involved.

What are the symptoms of a myocardial infarction?

The dominant symptom is cardiac pain as described in Chapter 3. The pain is typically in the middle of the front of the chest. It is similar to angina but lasts longer; somewhere between 20 minutes and 6 hours is the usual duration. A pain which is present continuously for more than 24 hours is unlikely to be produced by an infarction. It may be very severe and is often accompanied by sweating and anxiety. It is not altered by breathing or changes in position. Some breathlessness may also be noticed.

Contrary to a common belief, loss of consciousnesss is not a normal feature of a myocardial infarction. The pain can be so severe that the patient has to lie down and is temporarily unable to communicate. But he is still conscious. If he is really unrousable at this stage something more than a straightforward infarction has occurred or the diagnosis was incorrect. Few episodes of loss of consciousness are secondary to a myocardial infarction.

Who gets a myocardial infarction?

Angina and infarction both share the same basic problem of atherosclerosis of the coronary arteries. Infarction is less common than angina but they do affect similar people — usually men over 30 and women over 40 years. They share the same risk-factors (p.50). The increased risk of cigarette smokers is even greater for infarction than it is for angina.

Although both conditions affect a similar population they do not necessarily attack the same people. Many patients have angina without ever getting an infarction and vice versa.

Are infarctions produced by too much exertion?

No, they can occur at any time, even when resting in bed. As described above an infarction is produced by a sudden obstruction of coronary artery. The cells will be permanently damaged by the lack of blood regardless of the load on the heart at the time. Occasionally, an infarction does seem to be related to physical exertion. In these cases the damage was probably going to happen soon; the exercise was just the precipitating event.

Are they produced by stress?

Not as far as we know. Stress is very difficult to measure which hampers any research in the field. Once an infarction has occurred the patient and his relatives tend to look back for possible causes. Some form of stress can often be identified in the days leading up to the attack. But many of us have some stressful event in any period of a few days without developing an infarction. As yet no good evidence exists that stress precipitates heart attacks of any type, though its possible links with sudden death will be discussed later.

How is a myocardial infarction treated?

The essential features are pain-relief, rest and the treatment of any complications. A powerful painkilling drug, such as morphine or one of its derivatives given by injection, is required. These drugs work within minutes. If necessary further injections will be given. The mild sedation is a useful side-effect.

Complete rest is essential for the first few days. This often takes place in hospital. The damaged heart has to be allowed a short period of recovery with its output kept to a minimum. The rest is normally in bed though an occasional patient is more comfortable in a chair. At one time 6 weeks bed rest was recommended after an infarction. We now know that such a long period is not only unnecessary, but can also be harmful. Patients resting in bed for more than a few days are liable to a number of complications, such as clots in the veins and chest infections. Subsequent mobilization becomes more difficult as muscles become weak and joints go stiff. The standard treatment for a myocardial infarction is now a few days rest in bed followed by a gradual return to full activities.

How is the diagnosis made?

An infarction is only one of several possible causes for a severe pain in the chest. The diagnosis is often suggested by the character and duration of the pain, but tests are usually required to confirm it.

The electrocardiogram can be very helpful; one recording may be sufficient. Sometimes the changes are equivocal, so several recordings may be needed over the first few days to demonstrate progression of the abnormalities. The initial tracing can be normal but it is extremely rare for an infarction not to produce an abnormal electrocardiogram within a day or two.

Some patients have long-standing angina or previous infarctions. Their electrocardiograms may already be abnormal which makes confirmation of the diagnosis more difficult. Blood tests will be required. Damaged heart muscle releases chemicals known as enzymes which can be detected in the blood. But the enzymes will not reach diagnostic levels for a day or two. So blood samples are often taken for two or three days after a suspected infarction so that the enzymes can be measured.

An important practical point is that it can take several days before the diagnosis is confirmed or excluded. Doctors often have to treat the patient on the assumption that an infarction has occurred, but without definite confirmation. So patients may be admitted to a coronary care unit as a precaution, although the final conclusion is that the pain is not coming from the heart at all.

Why are some patients with infarctions admitted to coronary care units?

The basic treatment of an infarction, pain-relief and rest, is simple. But complications can occur in some patients and dealing with them may be more difficult. It is much better to anticipate problems and if possible prevent them occurring.

A coronary care unit allows close observation of patients, facilitating the prevention or treatment of any problems. The major complication in the first few hours after an infarction is an abnormal heart rhythm (arrhythmia). By monitoring the heart minor arrhythmias, of which the patient is unaware, can be detected. Their treatment will abort more serious rhythm problems. If major arrhythmias do occur, they can be dealt with promptly. The close observation also encourages the immediate treatment of heart failure or other complications,

Some patients do not need to be admitted to a coronary care unit. Rhythm problems mostly occur in the first few hours after an infarction. If admission has been delayed, the ordinary ward or even the patient's home may be more appropriate. The treatment available in the coronary care unit can also be used in the ordinary ward, though it may not be available as quickly.

How is the patient transported to hospital?

Ideally, he should be moved in an ambulance equipped and manned to deal with any rhythm problems that might occur during the journey. One solution is to provide a 'mobile coronary care unit' staffed by doctors and nurses. Another approach is to utilize specially trained ambulancemen. Both types of units are uncommon in the United Kingdom. Their benefits have been questioned as most journeys to hospital last only a few minutes and the incidence of serious complications in this short time is small. If 'resuscitation' ambulances are available (p.77) they can conveniently be used to transport patients with a suspected infarction to hospital.

What happens in a coronary care unit?

Most district hospitals in the United Kingdom have a coronary care unit. It may have a different name, such as cardiac monitoring unit, but the principle is the same. Sometimes it is combined with an intensive therapy unit for other medical problems.

The first aim in the unit is to relieve the pain and keep the patient rested and comfortable. The morphine or related drugs are given by intramuscular or intravenous injections. A small plastic tube may be left in an arm vein for the first couple of days so that drugs can be administered without delay. The pain-killing drugs may induce vomiting in a few unlucky patients; other drugs are often given at the same time to prevent this. Some drowsiness is another side-effect but this is helpful in keeping the patient rested for the first few hours. Coronary care units should be quiet and peaceful to help the patients feel as relaxed as possible. This minimizes the complications and helps the heart muscle to heal quickly.

The heart rhythm is monitored with the aid of wires attached to pads (electrodes) on the front of the chest. The display monitors may be on a central console or close to each bed. Any change in the rhythm can be detected immediately. Many such changes are trivial but if necessary drugs are administered into a vein, either as a single injection ('bolus') or a continuous infusion.

A few patients may develop a more serious arrhythmia. Parts of the heart muscle may try to beat in a very rapid, uncoordinated fashion. When this rhythm, which is known as ventricular fibrilliation, starts the ventricular muscle loses its ability to contract and relax. The pumping action of the heart is lost. Blood flow to the brain is cut off and unconsciousness follows within seconds. The rhythm must be treated immediately before the organs are seriously damaged by insufficient oxygenation. A direct current electrical shock across the chest (defibrillation) will abort this arrhythmia in nearly all cases if the shock is applied within a minute or so. After this the chances of success diminish. The prompt response is much easier to achieve in a coronary care unit.

The heart rate may be abnormally slow in the first few hours after an infarction. If necessary the rate can be speeded up with a temporary pacemaker (p.146). Many units have a small portable

X-ray machine so that the pacemaker wire can be inserted without moving the patient to the X-ray department.

In some coronary care units a simple right heart catheterization (p.37) can be performed without moving the patient from his bed. This sounds formidable but it can be done with surprising ease. A special tube (catheter) is inserted into a large vein with the aid of local anaesthetic. A small balloon is then blown up at the tip of the catheter. The blood stream takes the balloon and attached catheter into the right atrium, right ventricle, and pulmonary artery as required. The position of the catheter is determined by the pressure values; no X-ray equipment is needed. By measuring the pressures inside the heart the best treatment of any heart failure can be decided upon. The effects of the therapy can also be monitored.

What happens after leaving the coronary care unit?

A stay in the unit may last from a few hours to several days, depending on the circumstances. In many hospitals the determining factor is the time taken to find an empty bed on the ordinary wards! Gradual mobilization is now the plan. The speed at which this happens varies greatly from hospital to hospital. A common pattern, starting at the time of admission, would be about 3 days complete bed rest, followed by another 2 days sitting in a chair. Free mobility in the ward may be possible by the seventh to tenth day after admission. An unaccompanied patient might expect to be home within 2 weeks or less of the infarction. Women, and other patients who find it difficult to escape domestic duties, might go to some form of convalescence before returning home.

While in the ward the patients are still under observation but it is less intense than in the coronary care unit. The same facilities are available and treatment can be initiated promptly if necessary. But the aim is now to get the patient back to full active life and to reduce the risk of further heart problems. Treatment of high blood pressure can be initiated if necessary. Advice will be given about risk-factors, such as smoking and excess weight. Some patients may be started on low animal fat diets.

What happens after leaving the hospital?

Most patients return gradually to a normal life. Once again the speed varies greatly but many patients can aim to get back to unrestricted activities within 6 weeks of the infarction. This is the time to find out about any residual angina or heart failure so that they can be dealt with.

Many patients find the first few days at home very tiring. Even ambulatory patients in hospital expend very little energy as everything is on one level in a ward and close together. At home more activity is required. In addition the change from the 'safe' atmosphere of the hospital to the normal environment at home can produce anxiety, which makes any tiredness feel worse. This sensation is normal and passes within a few days.

Special exercise clinics are sometimes available. They usually involve supervised exercise in a hospital gymnasium. Although such clinics are by no means essential, they do give some patients the confidence to get back quickly to normal activities.

Even after a small infarction returning to normal life can be very difficult for a few people. A feeling of depression may persist for several months. Previously fit men may feel 'crippled' even though the heart is working quite normally. Recurrent, non-cardiac, chest pain can be a problem. Nearly all of us have pains in the chest at sometime, just as we have headaches or stomach ache. Under normal circumstances these pains are hardly noticed. But after an infarction, they seem much more important which in turn makes them worse. Most patients do not get these problems, but those that do have to work hard to regain their confidence and get back to normal.

Can a myocardial infarction be treated at home?

Although an acute infarction usually results in admission to hospital, home treatment is sometimes an alternative. Recent studies have shown that staying at home is perfectly acceptable in some patients. Indeed, there is a suggestion that some older patients may do better in their normal surroundings at home than in an unfamiliar hospital. It is only possible if there are no complications and the patient can be looked after. Opinions differ, but most experts feel that if the patient is seen within four hours of the onset of pain and a hospital is reasonably close, admission should be advised. If more than 4 hours have passed or the patient may take a long time to get to hospital, staying at home can be considered. The principles of treatment are the same whatever the location.

Should activities be limited after an infarction?

A permanent reduction of activities is rarely required after an infarction. Patients and their relatives are often very conscious of the possibility of precipitating a further episode by inappropriate exercise. But few infarctions occur during or soon after exertion, so this is an unnecessary fear. Indeed some evidence exists that regular exercise is beneficial in maintaining good health after leaving hospital.

So patients can expect to resume a full normal life once the convalescent period is over. This includes sex as well as work and leisure activities. But the resumption must be gradual. Over blown newspaper articles about men who run marathons after an infarction do not apply to everybody. Younger men can certainly take up running but the distance and speed must be increased gradually. Exercise which involves sudden effort such as lifting heavy weights or shovelling snow is less suitable and should be kept to a mimimum. This subject will be explored further in Chapter 8.

A few patients will find their activities limited by persisting angina or heart failure. Even then exercise should not be unduly curtailed. The permissible amount will vary but, in general, patients can be their own guide. If a patient can do something easily without symptoms, he should get on with it unless his doctor has advised otherwise.

Can driving be resumed after an infarction?

Most patients can return to driving a car once the acute phase is over. The precise timing depends on medical advice. In the United Kingdom the official recommendation is that car driving can normally be resumed 2 months after the infarction but the Licensing Centre must be notified.

The regulations are more strict for drivers of heavy goods vehicles and buses. Nobody with coronary artery disease is allowed to hold a licence for these vehicles. Bus and lorry drivers will have to find an alternative occupation. For similar reasons, pilots, both professional and amateur, are barred from flying, but most people can fly as passengers once the acute phase is over.

Does the heart pump normally after an infarction?

This depends on its size. Some heart cells are always destroyed by an infarction. Fibres form in the area of damage, producing firm scar tissue. A small to moderate sized infarction will not significantly affect the heart's pumping action though it will often leave residual abnormalites on the electrocardiogram. With a larger infarction the pumping action may be impaired. Heart failure could be produced but it will often be readily controlled by drug therapy.

Will the patient eventually develop another infarction?

In the months after discharge from hospital the patient is liable to hear graphic accounts of friends or neighbours who have had a series of infarctions. He may get the misguided impression that recurrence is inevitable. Unfortunately, the man who never has any more trouble does not make a good story. Many famous people have had a myocardial infarction in the past but remain active in public life today without any further problems. Their heart disease is rarely remembered for more than a year or two.

A long series of infarctions is the exception rather than the rule. With angina, the cells recover completely between the attacks so repeated pain is normal. With an infarction, the cells are permanently damaged and cannot produce any further trouble. A recurrence represents fresh coronary artery obstruction; another infarction is a possibility but it is by no means certain. Many people never have another. The risk can be reduced by preventative measures described in Chapter 8.

What drugs are used after an infarction?

Drugs may be used for a variety of purposes as described in the relevant sections of this book. Any residual angina or heart failure can be controlled. Hypertension should be treated. In the first few days sleeping pills are sometimes used to ensure rest at night. They should be stopped before the patient goes home from hospital to prevent long-term dependency.

For many years doctors have explored the possibility that drug therapy might decrease the risk of infarction, or at least minimize its effects if it occurred. Some false hope has been generated. But recent work has demonstrated that one group of drugs, beta blockers, can reduce the incidence of subsequent complications. These agents are also used in the treatment of angina, hypertension, and some abnormal rhythm. It is uncertain whether they act primarily by reducing the chance of another infarction or by preventing dangerous rhythms after the second infarction. Not all patients can take the drug for a variety of reasons, but in those that can they do reduce the number of serious complications in the first year after an infarction. We do not yet know whether the benefit continues for more than a year.

As a blood-clot precipitates an infarction, do blood-thinning drugs help?

Anticoagulant drugs inhibit blood clotting and are sometimes called blood-thinning drugs. Their popularity after an infarction has waxed and waned. The idea has some logic — reducing the risk of another clot in the coronary arteries should minimize the chance of another infarction. But trials have shown that the benefits are not great, probably because the drugs work better on veins than they do on arteries. The dosage of anticoagulant drugs such as warfarin has to be controlled by frequent blood tests and there is an appreciable incidence of unwanted bleeding. At the moment most doctors feel that the benefits do not outweigh the disadvantages sufficiently to recommend routine therapy, though particular patients may require long-term warfarin therapy.

Other drugs are being assessed to see whether their action of inhibiting clotting can prevent a further infarction. Warfarin influences the clotting ability of plasma, the liquid component of blood. These other drugs act on the platelets, very small cells in the blood which start the clotting mechanism. The platelets become less 'sticky' so they are less liable to clump together to form the nucleus of a clot. Aspirin has this effect in addition to its pain-relieving properties. Two other common 'antiplatelet' drugs are dipyridamole (Persantin) and sulphinpyrazone (Anturan). Their place in routine therapy is not yet decided though they can be helpful in some patients.

Does a heart operation help after an infarction?

If refractory angina is a problem, an operation to bypass the obstructed arteries with veins taken from the leg can control it (p.160). But the operation is not so effective in reducing the risk of further trouble and is done infrequently for this purpose in the United Kingdom. After an infarction the affected muscle is permanently damaged, so improving its blood supply will achieve nothing. In some people a fresh thrombus could compromise undamaged muscle; a vein graft should reduce the risk. But these patients are difficult to identify with certainty, even after cardiac catheterization. A few patients may be helped by an operation, but in the majority it seems that simple preventative measures and appropriate drug therapy are better than complex surgery.

What should you do if somebody may be having an infarction?

Severe, persistent, pain in the middle of the chest felt by a middle-aged or elderly man or woman may be a myocardial infarction. The victim should remain where he is and immediate medical advice should be sought. In the United Kingdom this will usually involve a general practitioner. He may be able to reassure the patient that the pain is not coming from the heart. But speed is important. Complications are commonest within an hour or two of an infarction, so urgent medical advice is essential. If the patient is away from home and a doctor cannot be found quickly, it may be best to call an emergency ambulance for immediate transport to a hospital accident and emergency department.

Until medical aid arrives the subject should be kept still and reassured that help is coming. A semi-recumbent or sitting position is better than lying completely flat. Calmness is essential. If the victim has some nitrate tablets designed to be placed under the tongue to relieve angina, two should be taken, one after another. Other, more long-acting, drugs may do more harm than good and extra doses should be avoided. Simple pain-relieving drugs, such as aspirin, are not usually powerful enough to get rid of the pain, but there is no harm in trying them.

Intermediate syndrome

What is the intermediate syndrome?

Not all episodes of cardiac pain can be neatly categorized as angina or a myocardial infarction. Sometimes the pain comes on at rest and persists, but permanent damage to the heart muscle does not follow. The syndrome is intermediate between the two conditions. The pain can last from a few minutes to several hours and often results in admission to a coronary care unit. It has a tendency to recur until satisfactory treatment is established.

As the definition of the syndrome has blurred edges, a number of terms have been used to describe particular aspects. Some contain assumptions about the risk of developing an infarction which are not warranted. Common terms are:

Acute coronary insufficiency
Pre-infarction angina
Pre-infarction syndrome
Unstable angina
Nocturnal angina
Angina at rest.

What produces the intermediate syndrome?

Once again, the cardiac pain is due to a shortage of blood flow to the heart muscle for the work required. In patients with the intermediate syndrome the blood flow is temporarily reduced by arterial thrombi or spasm. But the reduction is not sufficiently severe or prolonged to produce permanent damage. The muscle recovers.

How is intermediate syndrome diagnosed?

The character of the pain suggests that it may have a cardiac origin. This is confirmed by changes in the electrocardiogram. In the early stages it may be impossible to decide whether the patient is suffering from an infarction or the intermediate syndrome. The specific electrocardiographic changes or the nature of the pain may provide the answer later, but often an infarction is only excluded by absence of a significant rise in the blood's cardiac enzymes (p. 63).

The electrocardiographic abnormalities can be transitory and may only be present during the pain. If necessary the electrocardiogram can be monitored outside hospital with a portable tape recorder (p.30) to detect the changes. This method is also employed for atypical angina. Indeed, the main difference between the two conditions is that the atypical angina only lasts for a minute or two while the pain of the intermediate syndrome continues for longer.

Is the intermediate syndrome eventually followed by an infarction?

At one time it was thought that the syndrome was a common precursor of an infarction, hence the term 'pre-infarction angina'. But we now know that this is incorrect. Patients with the syndrome certainly do have a higher risk of infarction in the near future than those with stable angina. But in the vast majority, infarction does not follow the intermediate syndrome. No pattern of cardiac pain inevitably results in progression to an infarction; so the concept of a 'pre-infarction syndrome' is misleading.

How is the syndrome treated?

Although an infarction only develops in a minority, the potential risk demands careful, rapid treatment. Rest and pain relief are the first requirements. Admission to hospital is often needed because an infarction is suspected or because treatment can not be arranged at home. Doctors are justifiably cautious and will tend to treat the patient as if an infarction has occurred when they are in doubt.

Drugs used in the treatment of angina will help in the intermediate syndrome. A combination of drugs may be used to achieve rapid control. A reduction in the clotting ability of the blood (anticoagulation) can be helpful in some patients. This is done by an intravenous infusion of a drug called heparin, followed by warfarin taken by mouth. Appropriate advice will be given about reducing risk-factors as described in Chapter 8.

Is surgery indicated for the intermediate syndrome?

With rest and drug therapy the pain is normally controlled within a day or two. In a few patients the syndrome is resistant to therapy; either the pain keeps on returning after the first day or two, or further episodes occur weeks or months later. Coronary arteriography (p.39) is often indicated to see whether surgery will help. The operation is the same vein grafting procedure that is used to control angina. A few years ago it was sometimes performed within hours of admission, but it is now clear that the risks of surgery are increased in the acute phase, so rest and drug therapy are employed first. In selected patients a carefully planned operation can prevent a later myocardial infarction.

Sudden cardiac death

What is sudden cardiac death?

Heart disease is the commonest fatal illness in the developed world. Coronary artery disease is by far the most frequent cause of fatal heart disease, whether the death is sudden or not. The definition of 'sudden' has varied. In more leisurely times it referred to death within 24 hours of the onset of symptoms. Nowadays the common convention is that it has to occur within one hour to qualify. Some experts also include unwitnessed deaths in the definition.

Why is sudden cardiac death important?

Why is sudden cardiac death different from any other form of cardiac death? Non-sudden cardiac death represents the end of a period of deteriorating cardiac function. It is avoided by arresting the deterioration if possible, but even if this is achieved, a poorly functioning heart remains. With sudden cardiac death, the cause may be a transient rhythm disturbance. If it can be prevented, many years of normal cardiac function may follow.

The importance of sudden cardiac arrest has only been appreciated in the last few years. The old, incorrect, view was that an infarction was always the cause. The larger the infarction, the quicker the death. When a previously fit, middle-aged man dropped down dead, the problem was often described as a myocardial infarction or a 'massive heart attack'. Curiously, at a post mortem examination the pathologist could often find no evidence of an infarction, though the coronary arteries were usually diseased. The conventional view was that the death was so sudden that the pathological changes of an infarction had not had enough time to develop. The alternative explanation that no infarction had occurred was not seriously considered.

By the early 1970s defibrillation for ventricular fibrillation had become a common technique in coronary care units (p.65). Pumping of the blood ceases during ventricular fibrillation and it will always prove fatal unless it is reversed within a few minutes. It was then found that suitably equipped, mobile units could race through the streets and defibrillate people suffering from the arrhythmia outside hospital. This is not easy to achieve but it can be done with suitable organization. As a result several facts emerged. One was that ventricular fibrillation was the commonest terminal event in victims of sudden cardiac death. More importantly, the patients who were resuscitated would have died if special units had not got to them in time. In a sense they were survivors of 'sudden cardiac death' and could be investigated in detail later to find the underlying problem. The most interesting result was that at least half of the survivors had not developed an infarction at all.

The current view is that most examples of sudden cardiac death are produced by ventricular fibrillation. Some are secondary to a myocardial infarction, but it is not necessarily a large one. Many, perhaps the majority, do not have an acute infarction at all. If the patient is resuscitated from the ventricular fibrillation, the outlook may be many years of a normal, active life.

Is sudden cardiac death always the result of coronary artery disease ?

Not always, though about nine out of ten cases are. The remainder are secondary to other forms of heart muscle or valve disease.

Who is at risk of sudden cardiac death?

At the moment we are not very good at identifying those at risk. We know that certain groups of people, for example, heavy smokers and those with severe coronary artery disease, are more vulnerable; but even within these higher risk groups sudden cardiac death is a rarity. Certain severe rhythm problems in the past predispose to sudden cardiac death and require prophylactic treatment, though in a particular patient the chance of it occurring is not great.

One small section which has a high risk of sudden cardiac death is the group of patients who have been resuscitated from ventricular fibrillation occurring without an acute infarction. In the absence of long-term preventative therapy, the ventricular fibrillation would have a good chance of recurring. Chronic drug therapy is needed. But patients who have ventricular fibrillation at the time of, or soon after, a myocardial infarction do not have an increased risk of a later sudden cardiac death. It seems that in this latter group the rhythm disturbance is transitory and resolves with time.

What can be done to prevent sudden cardiac death?

This is an evolving subject. Rapid advances in our understanding of sudden cardiac death have been made in recent years. But therapeutic trials take time and the best method of prevention has not yet been agreed. Drugs used in treatment of ventricular arrythmias (p.141) can be taken long-term to abort threatened episodes of ventricular fibrillation. But this is a crude approach. As we cannot yet identify those at high risk, many have to take tablets for long periods, though in most the chance of a serious problem is small or non-existent.

An interesting topic which has surfaced recently is the possible role of acute psychological stress in the genesis of sudden cardiac death. Dying of fright may be a genuine entity. Coronary artery disease is the basic problem. But acute events, such as an argument, getting fired from a job, or being involved in a road accident, could be the final precipitating event in the few vulnerable people. A possible explanation for this would be the increased blood levels of catecholamines during acute psychological stress. Catecholamines are chemicals (hormones) produced by the body as part of its response to acute stress. High concentrations of catecholamines are known to precipitate ventricular fibrillation in some people. Occasionally, exhortations to 'keep calm and count to ten' might have some practical relevance. Chronic psychological stress is not important; a broken marriage or worry about housing does not disturb the heart rhythm.

What can be done to treat sudden cardiac death?

This may seem to be a curious question; by definition, death is untreatable. But we can rephrase the question — can ventricular fibrillation outside hospital be treated? The answer is yes. Special mobile units capable of getting to the patient within a few minutes are required. In a few areas of Britain the units are available, manned by trained ambulancemen or doctors. In many parts of the United States special 'paramedic' units are used to provide this emergency treatment. Once the ventricular fibrillation has been confirmed on an oscilloscope, a large electric shock is applied across the chest of the unconscious patient. The shock (defibrillation) often changes the fibrillation into a normal regular rhythm and the pumping action of the heart is restored. If necessary the shock is repeated. Normal cardiac resuscitation manoeuvres are employed to maintain the circulation until the rhythm has been corrected. Some of the ambulancemen or 'paramedics' are trained to use a small number of drugs to prevent the dangerous arrhythmias returning.

The feasibility of resuscitation from ventricular fibrillation in the community has not yet been generally accepted in the United Kingdom. Most experts feel that thousands of lives a year could be saved by the adoption of a national scheme. The costs would be small compared to many other life-saving procedures. But the concept is new and even the medical profession as a whole has not appreciated its full potential. Once it has been realized that people are dying unnecessarily, cardiac defibrillation out of hospital will gain more widespread support.

Cardiac resuscitation

Cardiac resuscitation is used for the treatment of cardiac arrest — complete cessation of the pumping action of the heart. Cardiac arrests can occur anywhere and all sorts of people may be called upon to react to the emergency that has happened in front of them. As we have seen, ventricular fibrillation is a common cause of cardiac arrest. Another is an absence of electrical activity which means that no contractions are being triggered (asystole). Cardiac resuscitation maintains the circulation until more definitive treatment, such as defibrillation, can be employed. Some cardiac arrests correct themselves spontaneously, but this is unlikely to occur once the ventricular fibrillation or asystole has been present for more than a minute. Resuscitation may also be needed for other emergencies, such as breathing difficulties or choking attacks; the modified techniques will not be dealt with here.

The best way to learn about cardiac resuscitation is to join a short teaching session. A variety of organizations hold them from time to time and reasonable proficiency can be obtained within two or three hours. Plastic models are used for practice. But not everybody is able to get to on of these training periods. So, in the belief that some form of resuscitation is better than nothing, the essentials will be described.

The first stage is to confirm the cardiac arrrest. The two features to look for are:

sudden loss of consciousness
cessation of breathing.

The victim should be shaken by the shoulder. 'Wake-up' should be shouted three times. Irregular breathing is common, part-icularly during sleep; cessation of breathing is being looked for. Those with sufficient experience can confirm that no pulse is present, but this may be difficult in the heat of the moment and should not delay resuscitation. Place the patient flat on his back on a firm surface and call for help.

The next stage is to open the airway into the lungs. Remove blood, vomit, loose teeth and broken dentures from the mouth, but leave well-fitting full dentures in place. Tilt the head back and pull the jaw upwards (Figure 4.4). This will open the airway and may allow breathing to start spontaneously. If it does not, artificial ventilation is required. Keep the patient's head tilted back and the jaw pulled upwards. Open the patient's mouth and pinch his nose. Take a deep breath, seal his mouth with yours, and breathe firmly into it. The breath should be enough to raise the patient's chest and no more. If the breath is difficult to get in, re-check the mouth and throat for obstructions.

If there are no signs of life after four breaths, cardiac massage will be needed unless a pulse can be felt. The technique of mouth-to-mouth ventilation may already be familiar as the 'kiss of life'. Although newspapers carry dramatic accounts of its success, *by itself* it is not a form of cardiac resuscitation. Cardiac massage is

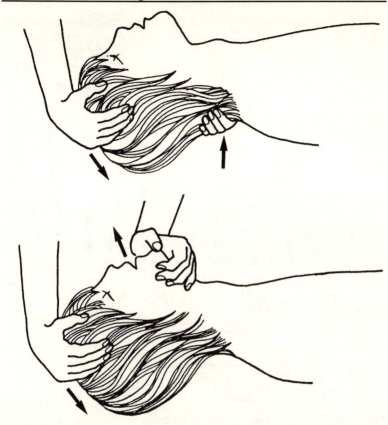

Figure 4.4. Cardiac resuscitation — positioning the head

required to move the blood around the body. To do this, place the heels of your hands, one on top of the other, over the lower half of the breastbone (Figure 4.5). Keeping your arms straight, lean forward and depress the breastbone by 4-5 centimetres. This should be repeated about once a second. If you are by yourself, do two lung inflations after every 15 second massages. With assistance, inflate the lungs after every 5 massages. At 2-minute intervals resuscitation should be briefly interrupted to check for spontaneous breathing and a pulse. If they have returned, the patient should be placed in the recovery position (Figure 4.6). Vomiting is common at this stage and this position will prevent the

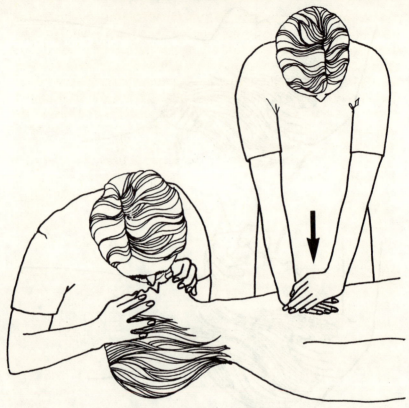

Figure 4.5. Cardiac massage and artifical ventilation

stomach contents getting into the lungs where they can do considerable damage in an unconscious patient.

Resuscitation should be stopped once breathing and a pulse have returned or when a doctor confirms that the situation is hopeless. Resuscitation aims to maintain the circulation but it rarely corrects the cardiac arrest. In some areas a special mobile unit, manned by doctors or ambulancemen, can be summoned to reverse the cardiac arrest. In other urban areas immediate transfer to hospital with continuing massage and ventilation is the best plan. In rural districts, finding a nearby doctor may be the best hope. Correction of cardiac arrest becomes more difficult as the minutes go by. The chances of success are small once resuscitation has been needed for more than ten minutes.

The dangers of cardiac massage in the absence of an arrest have been emphasized in the past, but the risks have probably been exaggerated. Such errors will be rare if it is remembered that the key features are sudden complete loss of consciousness and cessation of breathing. Cardiac massage does carry a small risk of damage to the chest wall or internal organs. But it should be noted that it is cardiac *massage*, not cardiac percussion. The chest wall should not be hit as hard as possible. Significant damage is rare and is outweighed by the lifesaving potential.

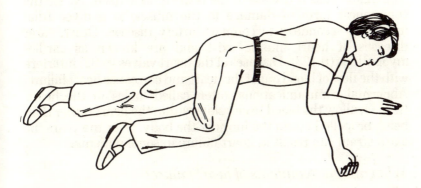

Figure 4.6. Recovery position

Heart Failure

Although heart failure has a number of possible causes, by far the commonest in the developed world is coronary artery disease; so the subject can be conveniently included in this chapter.

What is heart failure?

Heart failure is a concept that eludes a precise definition. The basic idea is that the failing heart is unable to pump sufficient blood for the needs of the body under all conditions. But the body's requirements vary tremendously; an old lady who is crippled by arthritis will make fewer demands on the heart than an athlete. An additional source of confusion is that the heart adapts to failure by increasing in size or by changing the pressures inside the heart. Some doctors confine the term to the acute phase, while others say that the heart is still in failure when adaptation has relieved the symptoms.

Heart failure is often a chronic problem rather than an acute event. The word 'failure' implies that something sudden, severe, and irrevocable has happened. But this is misleading; the circulation adapts to the heart failure and the process is often arrested. Many patients remain in well-controlled heart failure for years.

What produces heart failure?

The main cause is disease of the heart muscle itself. By far the commonest form of damage to the muscle is a myocardial infarction secondary to coronary artery disease. Other, rarer diseases of heart muscle exist and are known as cardio-myopathies (p.123). Diseases of the heart valves (p.92) interfere with the flow of blood out of the heart and can cause heart failure. Abnormal communications, often called 'holes in the heart' (p.111), allow the blood to circulate within the heart rather than being propelled out to the lungs or the body. Over the years the extra strain can result in heart failure in some patients.

What are the symptoms of heart failure?

The main symptoms are breathlessness, malaise, and fluid retention as described in Chapter 3. Heart failure itself is painless, though the underlying cause, such as a myocardial infarction, may hurt.

How is heart failure diagnosed?

As with many medical problems, the patient's symptoms will often suggest the diagnosis. The doctor then looks for signs that the heart is not pumping efficiently and fluid is being retained in the lungs or the rest of the body. He will inspect the veins in the neck to see whether they are engorged. He may feel the ankles for fluid retained under the skin. He will probably listen to the lungs with his stethoscope to hear the tiny crackling sounds produced by fluid. In addition the heart under strain produces extra sounds can sometimes be picked up. At the same time the doctor will be looking for the *cause* of the heart failure. Right heart failure, produced by problems in or around the right ventricle, is diagnosed by looking for signs of fluid retention in the neck veins or ankles. It is also known as congestive cardiac failure. Left heart failure, representing disease of the left heart, generates fluid in the lungs (pulmonary oedema). A chest X-ray is a good way of demonstrating this fluid. The two forms of failure often coexist. The initial left heart failure strains the right ventricle and eventually right heart failure follows.

Does heart failure deteriorate?

The answer to this question depends on the underlying problem. In general, the heart adapts well. If no fresh damage occurs, the failure will not deteriorate. Indeed, some spontaneous improvement can be expected. But sometimes the initial cause gets progressively worse, producing more heart failure. For example, a narrowed heart valve will often become more and more obstructed; only an operation can prevent increasing failure.

What is the treatment?

Rest

Rest is required until the failure is controlled. Depending on the severity of the failure, the rest may be strictly in bed or a chair, or just confinement to the house. Patients with left heart failure often find that they are more comfortable sitting up than lying down. They may prefer to sit, or even sleep, in a chair rather than stay in bed. Once the failure is treated normal activities can be resumed. Most patients can get back to a normal life, though some may have to accept some long-term restriction on their activities.

Diuretic tablets

'Water tablets' are often intial drug therapy. Diuretic tablets is the more correct description. Those in common use include frusemide (Lasic), bumetanide (Burinex), Navidrex and bendrofluazide. They promote an increased excretion of urine by the kidneys, reducing the amount of retained fluid which enables the heart to work more efficiently. Diuretic tablets are also used in the treatment of high blood pressure. A common misconception is that they are used to keep the kidneys working. In most patients the kidneys would function normally without them, though the failure might become worse. The start of diuretic therapy often results in an impressive volume of urine, but in the long-term a large output is not essential. Many diuretic tablets are designed to spread the increased urine production over the day so the patient does not notice it. With others the volume diminishes as the failure comes under control.

Diuretic tablets promote the excretion of potassium in the urine. This can deplete the body's potassium. Potassium is a mineral required for the functioning of several organs and, in severe cases, instability of the heart rhythm and muscle weakness in the limbs could follow. In many, but not all, patients on diuretic therapy the potassium depletion has to be corrected. One method is to give additional potassium by mouth. Some foods, such as fruit juices, bananas, prunes and potatoes, contain a high concentration of potassium and the diet can be modified accordingly. But it is difficult to be certain how much extra potassium the patient is taking by this means. Potassium-containing tablets can be used, either as a special slow-release tablet (Slow K) or for dissolving in water (Kloref). Some pharmaceutical companies have combined the potassium with the diuretic drug in one tablet; such preparations can often be recognized by 'K' after the name (Navidrex K, Burinex K, Hygroton K, etc.).

An alternative approach to controlling the potassium loss is to add in a rather different form of diuretic tablets which inhibit potassium excretion. This balances the potassium-losing effect of the initial drug. Diuretics which inhibit potassium excretion include spironolactone (Aldactone), amiloride (Midamor) and triamterene (Dytac). The two types of diuretics may be combined in one tablet (Moduretic, Dyazide, Aldactide).

Digitalis preparations

Digitalis preparations have been used in the treatment of heart failure for over 200 years. The original source was the foxglove. Nowadays synthetic preparations are used; digoxin (Lanoxin) is the most popular. Digoxin is particularly effective in failure which is accompanied by the irregular rhythm of atrial fibrillation (p.133). Indeed it is often given just for controlling that rhythm in the absence of failure. If the heart rhythm is regular, the benefits are less pronounced. Digoxin acts by increasing the force of heart muscle contraction. An important problem is that the effective concentration of the drug is close to the concentration that produces side-effects. So the patient and his doctor have to be alert for signs of toxicity. The first indication is often an unexplained loss of appetite, which can progress to nausea and vomiting. If the dose is not reduced, heart rhythm abnormalities may start to occur. The side-effects soon disappear once the dosage is adjusted.

Vasodilators

Some newer drugs, known as vasodilators, may be helpful in heart failure. They act by reducing the resistance to blood flow in the small vessels of the body. The failing heart then finds it easier to propel the blood around the body. Not suprisingly, they are also useful in reducing high blood pressures. At the moment vasodilator therapy is largely confined to patients resistant to other treatment, but this may change over the next few years. Drugs used in treatment of heart failure are summarized in Table 4.1.

Class	Common examples	Action	
Diuretic drugs	frusemide (Lasix) bumetanide (Burinex) cyclopenthiazide (Navidrex) bendrofluazide	removes retained fluid	standard therapy, well tolerated
Potassium supplements	Slow K Kloref	replaces lost potassium	often combined with diuretic
Potassium-retaining diuretics	amiloride (Midamor) spironolactone (Aldactone) triamterene (Dytac)	retains potassium and increases diuretic action	effective, costly
Digitalis preparations	digoxin (Lanoxin)	increases pumping action	easy to overdose, not always effective
Vasodilator drugs	hydralazine (Apresoline) prazosin (Hypovase)	reduces peripheral resistance	well tolerated, may be used more in the future

Table 4.1 Drugs used in the treatment of heart failure

Hypertension

Hypertension, or high blood pressure, is usually a variation on the normal rather than a disease. People have different blood pressures in the same way they have different heights and weights. Some have higher pressures than others. No natural division exists between 'normal' and 'abnormal' pressures. But we know that higher pressures are associated with certain diseases. A reduction in the pressure will abolish the extra risk of developing these problems. Hence the importance of identifying and controlling hypertension.

What causes hypertension?

In the vast majority of cases, hypertension is not a disease, so it does not have any particular cause. To look for a cause would be similar to asking why one person is 5 foot 10 inches tall and the next person is 5 foot 7. Like tallness, it does run in families to some extent, but many cases appear sporadically. Obesity will promote hypertension. Excessive salt intake may also be involved, though this is still controversial. Blood pressure tends to rise with age.

In a few patients the hypertension is an illness produced by a specific cause. The kidneys are involved in the regulation of blood pressure, so kidney disease can result in hypertension. This can be a difficult problem because the hypertension may worsen the kidney disease. Hormones, circulating messenger chemicals, are also concerned in the regulation of blood pressure. An excess of certain hormones can produce hypertension. Another cause is a severe narrowing of the aorta which is present from birth (coarctation). In order to push the blood past the partial obstruction, the pressure in the upper part of the body becomes elevated.

How is blood pressure measured?

A cuff is placed around the upper arm and inflated to a pressure above the blood pressure. This compresses the main artery in the arm. The cuff is connected to an instrument known as a sphygmomanometer (Figure 4.7). The pressure in the cuff forces mercury up a glass tube. The height of that mercury column in millimetres measures the pressure in the cuff.

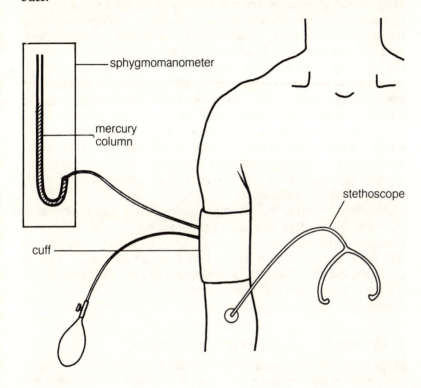

Figure 4.7. Blood pressure measurement

The doctor or nurse slowly releases the pressure in the cuff while listening with a stethoscope over the artery at the elbow. Once the cuff pressure is less than the maximum blood pressure (systolic pressure), the artery can open with each heart beat and a regular sound will be heard. When the cuff pressure is below the minimum blood pressure (diastolic pressure) the artery will be open all the time and the sounds disappear. The systolic and diastolic pressures are expressed together as the 'blood pressure'. A typical value might be 125/80.

What blood pressure is regarded as hypertension?

High blood pressures are not clearly separated from normal pressures. All we can say is that pressures over certain levels increase the risk complications such as strokes, heart disease, and kidney damage. The risks of developing these problems increase once the pressure is consistently over 140/90, so this is often taken as an arbitrary dividing line between normal and abnormal pressures. But the risks are minimal with a slight increase in pressure, and treatment has not yet been shown to be of benefit until the diastolic pressure is 105 millimetres or above. On whole the diastolic pressure is more reproducible and is an easier method of monitoring treatment than the systolic pressure. The correct management treatment of diastolic pressures in 90 - 100 range is still being debated.

Another problem in attempting to define hypertension is that the blood pressure alters throughout the day. A rise in pressure with exercise is normal. Even at rest, the pressures will vary, depending on how relaxed the subject is. It is quite common for the pressure to be elevated at the first visit to the doctor when the patient is anxious; subsequent readings can be all normal.

What are the symptoms of hypertension?

Hypertension produces no symptoms, though the complications of hypertension may do so. The elevation of pressure is often found when the patient is visiting a doctor for some other reason. It used to be thought that hypertension produced recurrent headaches. But we now know that these headaches are just as common in people with normal pressures.

Turning this question around, most people with hypertension will be unaware of it until the pressure is measured. So doctors will often take the opportunity to check the blood pressure during a visit to the surgery, although the patient's problem is unrelated. Unfortunately the first symptom of hypertension will be one of its complications, such as a stroke. A minute spent measuring the pressure can save a lifetime of disablement.

Does hypertension resolve spontaneously?

The blood pressure varies in everybody. An elevation one day may be followed by a normal pressure a few days later. But once the high pressure has been sustained for some time, it will rarely resolve spontaneously. In some patients weight loss, a reduction in the salt in their diet, or meditation controls the pressure, but in most cases drug therapy is required for a prolonged period.

What are the complications of hypertension?

Hypertension has its major effects on the arteries, the kidneys, and the heart.

The raised pressure inside the arteries promotes the formation of atherosclerosis. Untreated hypertension encourages coronary artery disease and poor circulation to the legs. The atherosclerosis may damage the brain arteries. The resulting obstruction or rupture of the artery can produce a stroke. .

The kidneys may also be damaged by hypertension. As we have seen kidney disease is a rare cause of the raised pressure. Conversely, any form of uncontrolled hypertension can worsen kidney function. The resulting damage to the kidneys can then make the hypertension worse. Fortunately drug therapy can be used to interrupt this vicious circle.

Apart from promoting coronary artery disease, the high blood pressure has direct effects on the heart muscle. The pressures inside the left ventricle also have to rise to maintain the flow of blood through the arteries. The muscle cells work harder to generate the increased pressures and the cells enlarge (hypertrophy). The heart muscle becomes thicker and so is more vulnerable to any deficiency in its blood supply secondary to coronary artery disease. In addition, the continuing strain on the heart will stretch the muscle, which can reduce the contractile force. The left ventricular cavity dilates and left heart failure follows. Until the final stage this process can be reversed by controlling the blood pressure.

The increased risk of strokes, kidney damage, and heart failure will be abolished by treatment of the hypertension. The danger of severe coronary artery disease is reduced, but not entirely eliminated, by lowering the pressure. This may be because the atherosclerosis of the coronary arteries has already occurred and cannot be easily reversed.

What is the treatment of hypertension?

Although drugs are often required, non-drug therapies have had some popularity in recent years. The benefits of losing weight have already been mentioned. With mild hypertension it may be all that is needed, but it is not always easy to achieve. A marked reduction in the salt content of food would help. But a very low salt diet is extremely unpalatable. Just avoiding salty foods and not adding extra salt at the tabl may help to some extent. Various forms of meditation, relaxation, and 'biofeedback' are in vogue. Many doctors are wary of such techniques, but the nervous system is involved in the control of everybody's blood pressure, so these methods of modifying brain function may be appropriate. They do seem to work at times. But they are unlikely to have a general application; the average patient would find the techniques difficult to master.

Drug treatment is the mainstay of therapy. The treatment will usually be continued indefinitely, so it is important that the drugs be free of side-effects and preferably only have to be taken once or twice a day. The common classes of drugs are listed below.

Diuretic drugs

Common examples: bendrofluazide, Navidrex K.

Other uses: heart failure.

Taken once daily and well-tolerated. Can precipitate gout or diabetes in a few people.

Beta blockers

Common examples: propranolol (Inderal), atenolol (Tenormin), oxprenolol (Trasicor), metoprolol (Lopressor, Betaloc).

Other uses: angina, abnormal rhythms, prophylaxis after myocardial infarction

Usually well tolerated but can worsen heart failure, asthma, and poor circulation. A few people have nightmares, tiredness,   or cold extremeties. Often the most effective drugs.

Vasodilators

Common examples: hydralazine (Apresoline), prazosin (Hypovase).
Other uses: heart failure.
Not very effective by themselves, but well tolerated and good in
  combination with other drugs for resistant hypertension.

Adrenergic blockers

Common examples: guanethidine (Ismelin), bethanidine (Esbatal).
Other uses: none.
Often produce an excessive drop in pressure on standing up.
  Not often used today.

Methyldopa

Methyldopa (Aldomat) is a drug which does not fit into other classes. It has no other uses. It is good at controlling moderate to severe hypertension when beta blockers cannot be used.

These drugs are preferred because they are effective and well tolerated, though any can produce side-effects in a few patients. Sometimes the symptoms are transitory and will disappear with continued treatment. If not, it is nearly always possible to find another drug, or combination of drugs, that will control the pressure without side-effects.

Hypertension in the elderly may not require any treatment. The studies which revealed the risks of high blood pressure concentrated on younger people. We have little information about the effects of high blood pressure in old age, but it often seems to be well tolerated. By contrast, drugs are not free of problems in this age group. Many doctors would hesitate about initiating anti-hypertension therapy in patients over 70 years old, unless one of the complications of hypertension was already present.

5

Other forms of heart disease

In recent years the public's interest in heart disease has largely focused on the various manifestations of coronary artery disease. These are certainly the commonest problems. But many other forms of heart disease can affect patients; some are quite frequent. It is a mistake to assume that 'heart trouble' means coronary artery disease.

This chapter will deal with heart disease which is not produced by narrowing of the coronary arteries. For clarity it will be divided into sections. But in real life, heart disease may resist this compartmentalization. Many patients will have more than one cardiac problem; for example, two heart valves may be affected, or a leaky valve may be accompanied by some coronary artery disease. Similarly, the division between heart disease in adults and in children can be artificial. A hole in the heart is commonly detected in childhood, but if it is not found the first symptoms may be felt in middle age. A general rule of medicine is that anything that could happen will happen occasionally, and this is particularly true of heart disease.

Valvular heart disease

As described on page 6 the heart has four valves. The right side of the heart contains the tricuspid valve between the right atrium and ventricle and the pulmonary valve between the right ventricle and the pulmonary artery. In the left side, the mitral valve is between the left atrium and ventricle and the aortic valve separates the left ventricle from the aorta. Valves are necessary to prevent the blood flowing backwards, which would make the heart's pumping action less effective. In general, each valve can be narrowed (stenosed), leaky (incompetent, regurgitant), or both narrowed and leaky. The importance of the valves varies. As we shall see, diseased mitral and aortic valves, which control the inflow and the outflow of the main pumping chamber, tend to produce more trouble than diseased tricuspid and pulmonary valves.

What causes heart valve disease?

Rheumatic fever

This illness can affect the heart in two ways. The acute illness, rheumatic fever, can temporarily involve the heart; but permanent damage is produced by the subsequent rheumatic heart disease which may follow years, or even decades, later.

Rheumatic fever is primarily a disease of children and young adults. It can occur in later life but then its effects are less serious and rheumatic heart disease does not follow. It starts as a throat infection due to a particular class of bacteria, the *Streptococcus.* Most streptococcal throat infections are brief, painful, affairs which respond quickly to penicillin and do not affect other organs. But a few children are more sensitive to the organism and a more generalized disease, rheumatic fever. follows a few weeks later. The organism is still confined to the throat but its effects are felt elsewhere. Rheumatic fever produces an arthritis which flits from joint to joint and gives the disease its name. Characteristic skin rashes may be seen. The uncontrolled writhing movements of St Vitus's dance are another manifestation. Abnormal noises (murmurs) may be heard from the heart valves, but these do not persist once the disease is finished. Rheumatic fever can be a severe illness, but a complete recovery usually follows.

But a few patients, particularly children with more than one attack of rheumatic fever, go on to develop rheumatic heart disease. This may not be apparent until several decades have passed. The exact mechanism is not understood but it seems that the insult to the valves produces changes which are undetectable at first. But the damage progesses slowly over the years until a fibrous reaction produces a stenosed or incompetent valve. The mitral valve is affected most often, followed by the aortic and tricuspid valves. The pulmonary valve is not affected to any significant extent.

Sixty years ago rheumatic fever was a common problem; now it is rarely seen. This improvement is partly due to better social conditions which make children less vulnerable to bacterial infection and reduce their spread. Another reason is the introduction of antibiotics 40 years ago. Streptococcal throat infections can be controlled quickly before any other organs are affected. A child who has rheumatic fever will often be placed on continuous low-dose penicillin therapy to prevent a second attack. The development of rheumatic heart disease usually requires multiple episodes of rheumatic fever.

But in spite of the decline in rheumatic fever, rheumatic heart disease is still important. The greater incidence of the acute illness 50 years ago is still having an effect today. Rheumatic fever remains common in less developed parts of the world, whose inhabitants may have moved to developed countries before the chronic valve damage is apparent. Mild attacks of rheumatic fever are difficult to distinguish from an ordinary throat infection or another feverish illness of childhood. Some examples of valve damage seem to be secondary to mild episodes which were not diagnosed at the time. The extinction of rheumatic heart disease has been predicted for 20 years. But, although its incidence has declined, hopes of a complete disappearance are premature.

Congenital deformities

One or more valves may be formed incorrectly while the baby is developing inside the womb. These congenitally deformed valves can be stenosed or incompetent. The adjective congenital does not mean that the defect is inherited, though it can be occasionally. Athough the deformed valve is present at birth, it may not be detected for several years, perhaps not until adulthood. Stenosis of the pulmonary or aortic valves and incompetence of the mitral valve are the commonest congenital valve deformities. The subject will be discussed later along with other forms of heart disease in children.

Degeneration

Heart valves are remarkably reliable. In many people they work at least 60 times a minute for over 70 years. Although the man-made valves that are inserted at operation are good, they are not as tough as natural valves.

But in a few people the natural valves do not last for a whole lifetime. They start to deteriorate. This degeneration particularly affects the aortic and mitral valves. The aortic valve becomes heavily calcified, producing progressive stenosis. If the valve already has a mild congenital deformity, the calcification may start in middle age. With the mitral valve, the degeneration leads to stretching of the valve. The two halves of the mitral valve no longer fit together and the valve is now incompetent.

Prolapsing mitral valve

Functionally, the mitral valve is made up of two 'leaflets', which can be likened to two half parachutes (Figure 5.1). During diastole when the blood is flowing through the valve into the left ventricle, the parachutes are collapsed down. In systole, the raised pressure in the left ventricle fills up the

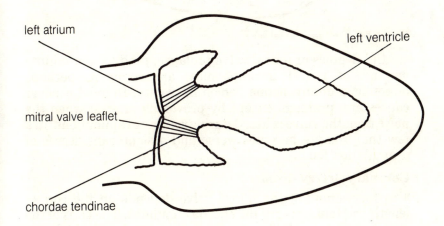

Figure 5.1 The mitral valve.

95

parachute canopies and they slam shut, preventing the blood from flowing back into the left atrium as the ventricle contracts. The shape of the valve is maintained by fibrous strands known as chordae tendinae. They are the equivalent of the cords of a parachute.

If these fibrous strands are too long, the ventricular contraction will force the valve leaflet back into the left atrium (Figure 5.2). This is known as a prolapsing mitral valve. The two leaflets are no longer closely applied to each other and some mitral incompetence will result. The cause of the excessive length of the chordae tendinae is uncertain. It could be a congenital deformity which is often not noticed until adulthood.

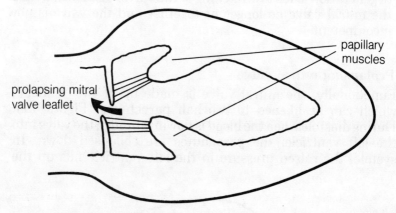

Figure 5.2. Prolapsing mitral valve

Mild degrees of mitral valve prolapse, producing a minute amount of mitral incompetence, are common, perhaps affecting as many as one person in twenty. In most it never causes any problem, except by provoking interest when the noise from the valve is heard during routine examinations. In a few the prolapse becomes worse and a significant degree of regurgitation follows.

Coronary artery disease

The functioning of the mitral valve depends on the correct length and tensioning of the chordae tendinae. The ends of the chordae are attached to two papillary muscles which are muscular protuberances from the wall of the left ventricle. Like the rest of the ventricular muscle, the papillary muscles are vulnerable to the oxygen shortage produced by coronary artery disease. They can be involved in a myocardial infarction. The damaged papillary muscles will no longer be able to maintain the correct tension on the chordae tendinae. As a result, the edges of the two mitral valve leaflets will not be held firmly together as the ventricle contracts and incompetence will occur.

Ventricular dilatation

In heart failure (p.82) the ventricles dilate in order to maintain the blood flow to the lungs and the rest of the body. The dilatation primarily involves the ventricular muscles but it can also stretch the fibrous ring which supports the mitral or tricuspid valve. The enlarged ring means that the valve leaflets no longer come together during ventricular contraction. Valve incompetence is the result.

So a failing left ventricle may stretch the mitral valve ring. The mitral incompetence will make the heart failure worse. The tricuspid valve has a similar structure to the mitral valve. So a right ventricle which is under strain will dilate and tend to produce tricuspid incompetence.

Connective tissue disease

Connective tissue is the name given to the cells, often fibrous in type, which are between the more specialized cells. The specialized cells deal with particular functions, such as contraction or excretion of urine. The connective tissue cells provide strength and keep the other cells correctly orientated, but they do not have specialized functions.

A number of problems can affect the connective tissue and they are grouped together under the term 'connective tissue disease'. Not suprisingly, a variety of organs can be affected. For example, the joints may be lax or the lens of the eye can be displaced. In particular, the strength of the heart valves may be reduced. The valve is then stretched by the pressures inside the heart and major blood vessels, and incompetence will follow. The aortic valve is the commonest valve to be affected, but the mitral may also be involved. Connective tissue disease is rare. One of the best-known forms is Marfan's syndrome where aortic and mitral valve deformities accompany abnormally long limbs and dislocations of the lenses of the eyes.

Syphilis

Before the discovery of penicillin syphilis was a fairly common cause of aortic valve incompetence. Now it is extremely rare.

An infection inside the heart (endocarditis) and a disruption of the wall of the aorta (dissection of the aorta) can also produce valve damage. They will be discussed later in this chapter.

What are the different types of valve disease?

For clarity, each problem will be considered separately, but they often occur in combination. Most valve deformities are too mild to produce any symptoms.

Aortic stenosis

Causes: congenital, rheumatic, degenerative.
Common symptoms: chest pain, breathlessness, dizziness on exertion.
Often the only valve problem. Mild examples are asymptomatic and are often discovered by chance.

Aortic incompetence

Causes: congenital, rheumatic, degenerative, connective tissue disease, syphilis.
Common symptoms: chest pain, breathlessness.
Can occur by itself or with aortic stenosis.

Mitral stenosis

Causes: rheumatic, rarely congenital.
Common symptoms: breathlessness, tiredness, palpitations.
Sometimes the only valve problem. Commoner in women than men.

Mitral incompetence

Causes: congenital rheumatic, degenerative, coronary artery disease, ventricular dilatation, prolapsing leaflet, connective tissue disease.
Common symptoms: breathlessness, tiredness.
Mild forms due to a prolapsing leaflet are so common that they can hardly be regarded as abnormal. More severe mitral incompetence can complicate many forms of heart disease.

Pulmonary stenosis
Cause: congenital.
Common symptom: tiredness.
Often a trivial problem.

Pulmonary incompetence
Cause: usually secondary to raised pressure in the pulmonary artery (pulmonary hypertension, p.128).
Common symptoms: none.
The incompetent pulmonary valve does not produce symptoms, though the cause of the raised pulmonary artery pressure may do so.

Tricuspid stenosis
Causes: rheumatic, congenital.
Common symptoms: peripheral fluid retention, tiredness.
Rheumatic tricuspid stenosis is always accompanied by rheumatic mitral or aortic valve disease.

Tricuspid incompetence
Causes: ventricular dilatation, rheumatic, congenital.
Common symptoms: peripheral fluid retention, tiredness, pulsation in the neck.
Most examples are due to ventricular dilatation in right heart failure.

What produces the symptoms of valve disease?

The symptoms are not specific to valve disease and are discussed in Chapter 3. For example, the heart pain of aortic stenosis is the same as the pain produced by coronary artery disease. With the narrowed valve the left ventricle thickens to provide the necessary force to drive the blood through the obstruction. The oxygen demands of the muscle outstrip its blood supply and pain is felt. With mitral stenosis the pressure in the left atrium rises to force the blood through the narrowing into the left ventricle. But the raised pressure increases the amount of blood in the lung vessels. Some of the blood fluid will leak out into the lungs and produce breathlessness. The symptoms are similar whether the excess fluid in the lungs (pulmonary oedema) is the result of heart failure or mitral stenosis.

How is valve disease diagnosed?

Unlike coronary artery disease which is mainly diagnosed from the patient's story, physical examination is the key to valve disease. Deformed valves produce noises (murmurs) which can be heard with a stethoscope. In addition, other findings on examination are associated with particular valve disorders. A fairly confident 'bed-side' diagnosis can usually be reached, though investigations are sometimes needed to confirm it and to assess the severity.

Murmurs

Murmurs are blowing noises of variable intensity. They are produced by turbulence in the blood stream, either by increased flow across a normal valve or by normal flow across a diseased valve. Some are due to blood regurgitating through an incompetent valve or crossing an abnormal communication such as a hole in the heart.

Murmurs may be heard in systole when the ventricles are contracting (systolic murmurs) or during diastole when the ventricles are filling from the atria (diastolic murmurs). Some are specific; a murmur heard in the middle of diastole is normally due to blood flow across a narrowed mitral or triscuspid valve — mitral or tricuspid stenosis. Others have a greater number of possible causes and the additional findings on examination must be interpreted carefully for a correct diagnosis. The noise from a particular valve will tend to be the loudest in one area of the chest surface and this can be useful in establishing a diagnosis.

Pulse

Some other findings are characteristic of particular valve problems. For example, tricuspid incompetence produces a typical pulsation in the neck veins which is diagnostic by itself. The incompetent valve allows the contraction of the right ventricle to force blood back through the right atrium and up into the veins. With aortic incompetence, some of the blood that flows out into the aorta leaks back into the left ventricle through the incompetent valve. This produces a 'collapsing' feel to the pulse as the blood returns to the ventricle; it is very suggestive of aortic incompetence.

Electrocardiogram and X-ray

The electrocardiogram (p.23) and the chest X-ray (p.22) are of some help in diagnosing valve disease. For example, calcification of the aortic or mitral valve seen on a sideways chest X-ray is an indication of degeneration of these valves. But they are often more useful in assessing the *severity* of any valve damage. The problem is diagnosed by physical examination and then the chest X-ray and electrocardiogram are helpful in deciding how bad it is. One example is the characteristic changes in the electrocardiogram induced by increasing severity of aortic stenosis. Another is the progressive enlargement of the heart shadow on a chest X-ray secondary to worsening mitral incompetence.

Echocardiogram

In recent years the echocardiogram (p.32) has become available in many hospitals for the detection and confirmation of valve disease. The movement of the aortic and mitral valves can usually be seen with every test and other valves can often be detected. With some valve problems the echocardiogram is very accurate. A normal picture of the mitral valve excludes any significant mitral stenosis. A diagnosis of mitral valve prolapse can often be only made confidently with the help of an echocardiogram. But other valve abnormalities have less specific appearances and the findings of the test have to be interpreted in conjunction with the physical examination. The echocardiogram does have the advantage of causing no discomfort and so it is readily repeated.

If a murmur is heard does that mean that valve disease is present?

No, it does not. Murmurs are common, most of them do not represent any heart disease though a few do. They are particularly numerous in children; careful listening may reveal a murmur in about one child in five. Murmurs are also heard in some adults with a normal heart. A little turbulence in the blood is not unusual. Anything that make the heart pump harder, such as exercise or pregnancy, will increase the turbulence and make the murmur louder. Some people have a narrow front to back diameter of the chest; this brings the heart closer to the chest wall and any turbulence will be heard more easily.

The main problem with these 'innocent' or 'flow' murmurs is that heart disease may be suspected when none exists. Difficulties with applications for jobs or life insurance may follow. If there is doubt about the significance of a newly discovered murmur, a detailed assessment will often prevent trouble later.

Does valve disease improve spontaneously?

In general it does not, though there are a few exceptions. The heart has some capacity to adapt but the valves themselves are largely inert fibrous structures and the body is unable to repair them. One exception is an incompetent mitral or tricuspid valve secondary to ventricular dilatation. If the dilatation can be reduced, the incompetence should improve. Another exception is mitral incompetence produced by an infarction of the papillary muscles; as the infarction heals the incompetence may diminish. But the vast majority of valve problems persist indefinitely, although treatment can control the symptoms.

Does valve disease progress?

Some valve abnormalities remain unchanged for decades while others progress more quickly. Disease which is secondary to rheumatic heart disease or degeneration often worsens over the years. Unfortunately, it is difficult to predict which problems are going to remain static and which will become worse. Many are unaltered for the whole of the patient's life, some worsen gradually over several years, and a few deteriorate rapidly. A doctor will often want to see a patient with valve disease at regular intervals so that any progression can be detected.

What are the complications of valve disease?

Atrial fibrillation

One complication is an irregular heart rhythm (atrial fibrillation), particularly with mitral stenosis. Due to the stenosis the blood cannot pass easily fron the left atrium to the left ventricle. The pressure in the left atrium rises to force the blood through the narrowed valve and eventually the increased pressure may strain the muscle of the atrial wall. The muscle will then become fibrous. The increased size of the left atrium and the presence of electrically inert fibrous areas means that all the atrium may not be excited with each heart beat (p.10). The electrical activity in the atrium becomes uncoordinated and atrial fibrillation (p.133) follows. The irregular atrial contraction will trigger disorderly ventricular activity, producing an irregular pulse.

Regular contraction of the left atrium helps to push the blood through the stenosed mitral valve. At the onset of atrial fibrillation this action will be lost and symptoms may worsen in some patients. However, this is only a temporary phenomenon and the heart adapts to the irregular rhythm. Chronic atrial fibrillation is a normal feature of long-standing mitral stenosis.

Aortic stenosis may strain the left ventricle in the same manner as mitral stenosis straining the left atrium. Similarly the regular rhythm of the ventricle may be replaced by intermittently abnormal rhythms if the stenosis is severe. This may be the cause of worsening symptoms.

Blood clots

Another complication of mitral stenosis is the release of blood clots into the circulation. The clots are known as emboli once they are in the circulation and the process is called arterial embolization. With the stenosis the blood pools in the left atrium and the stagnant blood is an ideal site for clot formation. The clots are unimportant while in the left atrium. But if they break off to become emboli, major complications can occur. The emboli will travel in the blood stream until the arteries become so small that the clots get stuck. The embolus will then block the vessel, drastically reducing the blood flow to whatever organ the artery is supplying. If the embolus lodges in the brain, a stroke may follow. A gangrenous leg could be produced by obstruction of blood flow to the lower extremities. Other organs commonly affected are the kidneys and the bowel.

The drastic effects of some emboli may be alleviated by prompt treatment, but the damage can be irreversible. The best treatment is to prevent blood clots forming in the left atrium. The combination of mitral stenosis and atrial fibrillation is usually treated with long-term anticoagulant drugs, such as warfarin, which inhibit clotting (coagulation). Some patients with mitral stenosis and a normal regular rhythm also need warfarin therapy. This treatment is a nuisance, as frequent blood tests are required to check that the dosage is correct, but it is well worthwhile to prevent the potentially serious complications of arterial embolization. Warfarin is also used as a rat poison. But the doses are much, much higher and the rats do not have any blood tests.

Is valve disease dangerous?

We have already seen that some people can have a noise from a valve (murmur) without any abnormality being present. Others have a trivial valve deformity which is not causing any problems and never will do. In some the trivial deformity will get worse, producing symptoms but without any real danger.

But a few patients develop serious valve deformities which can be dangerous. As mentioned above, severe aortic stenosis can produce serious ventricular arrhythmias. In addition severe stenosis or incompetence of a valve can place a chronic stress on the right or left ventricle. In the last resort the heart may be unable to pump enough blood, either because the valve disease has become so severe or because the ventricular muscle is damaged by the chronic strain.

But these dangers do not develop overnight. They are usually at the end of a long period of deterioration. Nowadays the process is commonly arrested by drugs or surgery before this late stage.

What is the treatment of valve disease?

Most patients with valve disease do not require any treatment except advice about preventing endocarditis (see below). Warfarin therapy is often needed for those with mitral stenosis to stop embolization from the left atrium (see above). A few patients will require drugs to control heart failure induced by valve disease. This treatment is along standard lines with diuretic therapy, digoxin, and vasolidator drugs (p.83). Anti-arrhythmic drugs could be needed for the control of abnormal rhythms (p.140).

Nowadays surgery is the mainstay of the treatment for severe valve disease in all except the elderly. The valves can sometimes be repaired but replacement with an artificial valve is often needed. This will be described in Chapter 7.

When is surgery needed?

Sometimes surgery is performed to control heart failure. On other occasions an operation may be required to prevent further strain on the ventricle or because serious arrhythmias might occur. Occasionally, these prophylactic operations may be done before the patient has developed any symptoms.

The timing of surgery for heart failure is relatively easy. If the failure is not controlled by drugs, detailed investigations are performed. They may indicate that the reduced heart output is largely due to the diseased valve. Unless the patient has other medical problems, an operations will then be the best form of treatment.

The decision about when to operate on a heart valve prophylactically is much more difficult. This is particularly true with a diseased aortic valve. If the operation is left too late, the left ventricle may already be permanently damaged and the end result is poor. If it is done too early, the patient may have been exposed to the discomfort and risk of an operation without any benefit. No single feature in the patient's story, examination, or tests can indicate the best time for operation.

When is cardiac catheterization required?

Cardiac catheterization (p.37), is carried out when surgery is being considered; it is not needed for diagnostic purposes. The test measures the severity of a valve defect. The information helps to determine whether an operation is the best treatment and also the best type of operation. Cardiac catheterization is not required before every valve operation; sometimes all the necessary information can be obtained from simpler tests. Conversely, a few patients will need more than one catheterization at intervals of a few years to find the best time for surgery.

Can valve disease be prevented?

Apart from mitral incompetence secondary to a myocardial infarction, the risk-factors which are involved in the genesis of coronary artery disease are not responsible for valve abnormalities. In general, little can be done to prevent valve disease. An exception is the avoidance of rheumatic fever which may go on to rheumatic heart disease. We have already seen how the incidence of this acute illness has been reduced by better social conditions and the availability of antibiotics for throat infections. Rheumatic heart disease usually follows *two or more* attacks of rheumatic fever in childhood. So children who have one attack are normally placed on continuous low-dose penicillin therapy until they leave school to prevent a second attack.

A few other causes of valve damage can be avoided. Syphilis can be treated with penicillin, but it is very rare today. German measles in early pregnancy can produce certain congenital valve deformities; this is one of the reasons for the routine immunization against German measles for all girls.

Endocarditis

What is endocarditis?

Endocarditis is an infection inside the heart. It can be known as infectious endocarditis (IE), bacterial endocarditis (BE), or subacute bacterial endocarditis (SBE). Although the large majority of cases are produced by bacteria, some are due to moulds or other organisms, so the general term infectious endocarditis or just endocarditis is preferable. It is extremely rare for a normal heart to be affected by endocarditis. The infection attacks diseased valves or other abnormal structures in the heart. The initial deformity may be trivial but it still could be a site for endocarditis. Once established the bacteria are difficult to eradicate. The heart valves are made of inert fibrous material without blood vessels. The bacteria hide in the valves or other cardiac structures away from the antibiotics in the blood stream.

Why is endocarditis important?

One hazard of endocarditis is that the infection may be difficult to control. It is rarely an acute infection like pneumonia or gastroenteritis. Endocarditis normally develops slowly with rather mundane symptoms, such as tiredness or a mild fever, whose significance is often missed in the early stages. By the time the diagnosis is made by growing the bacteria from the blood, the infection is well established and difficult to eradicate. It can have widespread toxic effects. In addition, collections of fibres and blood cells, called vegetations, can form at the site of the infection. The vegetations can break off into the blood stream to form emboli in a similar manner to the blood clots from the left atrium in mitral stenosis. These emboli have the same effects as those in mitral stenosis (see above), but differ in not being preventable by warfarin therapy. Endocarditis can be a very serious infection.

Another complication of endocarditis is that the affected heart structure suffers further damage. The preinfection abnormality may be minimal but some deterioration will always follow. It may be slight and not merit any further treatment. At times it is severe and surgery may be required. As we have seen, heart valves have no significant capacity to repair themselves, so any damage is permanent.

What heart structure can be involved in endocarditis?

Most examples of valve disease and holes in the heart or other congenital deformities can be affected, though the degree of risk varies considerably. One type of hole in the heart, secundum atrial septal defect, is never the site of endocarditis. Deformities which produce a high pressure jet of blood through a small hole, such as aortic regurgitation, are more at risk. Endocarditis is not common with any heart abnormality, but its potential seriousness means that vigilance is needed. In general, patients whose only heart problem is coronary artery disease do not get endocarditis.

How is endocarditis treated?

In about four cases out of five, the diagnosis is first established by finding the infectious organism in the blood. To do this, the blood is incubated in a culture bottle, allowing the small number of organisms to multiply. After a few days the numbers are sufficient to be seen under the microscope. The infectious agent is tested for its sensitivity to various antibiotics so that the best treatment can be selected. In the remaining patients, the diagnosis is suspected but an organism cannot be detected. Then the antibiotic treatment will have to be 'blind'.

The antibiotics are given for 4 to 6 weeks or even longer. Hospital admission is essential. A high blood concentration must be obtained so that the antibiotic can diffuse into the fibrous valves and eradicate the organisms lurking there. The doses are much higher than those employed for common infections such as pneumonia. Initially, the antibiotics are often given directly into the veins. The therapy is long and tedious but essential to eliminate the infection. Before the discovery of antibiotics the disease was nearly always fatal. Nowadays it will be cured if sufficient care is taken.

Surgery is necessary for a few patients. Some organisms, particularly certain moulds, can be checked by antibiotic therapy but are not eradicated. Surgical correction of the underlying deformity may be the only way of avoiding a chronic debilitating infection. More commonly an infected valve may become severely incompetent as a result of the endocarditis. If possible the infection is controlled first but a valve-replacement operation can be performed at any stage to avoid dangerous heart failure.

How is endocarditis prevented?

The first stage is to identify patients at risk. Almost anybody with valvular or congenital heart defects could develop endocarditis though there are one or two exceptions. Coronary artery disease is not complicated by endocarditis.

The basic mechanism is that organisms get into the blood and then, in a few people stick to the deformed heart structures, initiating the infection. The bacteria in the mouth are the main source of organisms. All our mouths are colonized

by bacteria which do not produce any infection if th
there. But once they get into the blood, they may lodg
heart to produce endocarditis. Entry into the blood i
any dental procedure which produces bleeding, such
extractions or vigorous descaling. If the blood can get out,
bacteria can get in. When dental hygiene has been neglected,
many more bacteria are present and they can be released into
the blood just by chewing food.

So patients at risk from endocarditis need a dental
inspection and any necessary cleaning every 6 months. It's
good for the teeth as well! The dentist needs to know about the
risk of endocarditis. He will give an antibiotic about an hour
before any procedure which might induce bleeding, so that any
bacteria leaking into the blood are eliminated. Some other
surgical operations, particularly those in the bowel or bladder,
could also allow bacteria to gain access to the blood. The
patient should tell the surgeon about the heart; a trivial
roughening of a valve will not be relevant to the performance of
the operation, but it is still a potential site of infection. An
appropriate antibiotic will be given.

Heart disease in children

No hard division exist between heart disease in children and in
adults. Most problems that affect adults can occasionally
occur in children and vice versa. But in adults the emphasis is
on coronary artery disease, while in children this is rarely
encountered and the main problems are congenital deformities, that is, deformities present at birth. This section will
largely be concerned with these congenital abnormalities. But it
should not be forgotten that children can also acquire heart
disease. In particular, endocarditis is a significant risk in older
children.

What causes congenital heart disease?

A baby's heart is formed within the first three months of pregnancy. It starts off as a simple tube which is twisted and part-
itioned to form the four chambers, valves, and associated
vessels. If the process is not completed correctly, a congenital
defect will result. Almost any step can go wrong occasionally,

though some defects are much commoner than others. Sometimes the congenital heart disease is associated with other non-cardiac abnormalities. For example, children with Down's syndrome ('mongolism') often have holes in the heart.

In at least nine cases out of ten no specific reason for the heart defect can be found. In the remainder a cause can be identified. Maternal thalidomide therapy has produced heart defects. German measles in the first 3 months of pregnancy is another cause, though this is rare since the advent of protective immunization and legal abortions. A problem that has aroused recent interest is excessive alcohol intake in early pregnancy; it also seems to be associated with heart defects in the baby.

Is congenital heart disease inherited?

Inheritance has a minor role, but it is rarely the major factor. With a fairly common problem such as congenital heart disease, by chance two members of the same family might be involved. It does seem that two relatives are affected more often than the rules of chance would predict. But most cases occur at random. This is well illustrated by identical twins, who share the same inheritance: normally only one twin has the congenital heart defect. Many congenital heart defects *can* occur in a familial form which affects most generations. However, they are rare.

Parents who have had one affected child often ask whether their next baby will have heart disease. Specialist genetic advice may be needed if the heart defect is known to run in families. Otherwise the risk that the next baby will be affected is less than one in 25.

Is congenital heart disease common?

About 0.8 per cent of all babies have some form of heart abnormality though in many cases it is trivial. This figure may be an underestimate, as some problems, such as minor valve abnormalities, may not be discovered till adult life. Heart disease is one of the commonest types of congenital malformation. Overall boys are more affected, though some conditions are commoner in girls.

Why are children often affected so soon after birth?

This may seem a ridiculous question. If a baby has a serious cardiac problem, the first few days of life would seem to be the obvious time for it to cause trouble. But, in one sense, the baby is already 9 months old at birth. So the question could be put — why does the baby grow normally in the mother's womb but run into difficulties soon after birth?

Babies are affected in this way because the circulation changes at birth. Inside the womb no air is entering the lungs. The baby's oxygen is obtained from the mother's blood through the placenta. The baby's blood bypasses the unused lungs. At birth the lungs are inflated and the circulation is adjusted so that all the blood flows through the lungs before being pumped around the rest of the body. This is the normal adult arrangement. Many defects in the heart are unimportant while the baby is inside the womb, but then cause trouble once the circulation has adapted to its normal form. The changeover takes several hours, so a baby can be healthy at birth but then become ill with heart disease a few hours later.

What are the types of congenital heart disease?

The number of potential defects is enormous, but the common ones can be divided into three categories — shunts, obstructions, and complex defects. Combinations of defects often occur.

Shunts

A hole in the heart or other abnormal communication will allow blood to flow (shunt) from the higher pressure left heart into the right heart. In other words the blood will circulate within the heart, wasting some of the pumping action.

Atrial septal defect (ASD)

This is a persistent hole between the two atria. It occurs in two forms — *primum* which is associated with other defects and *secundum* which often occurs in isolation. A secundum defect is commoner. A small secundum defect is a trivial problem and requires no treatment. If it is moderate sized no symptoms are produced in childhood, but in middle age complications may develop; so closure is often advised at a convenient time in adolescence. A large defect may need an earlier operation.

Ventricular septal defect (VSD)

A hole between the two ventricles is the commonest congenital heart defect (Figure 5.3). Fortunately it will often close spontaneously in the first few years of childhood. Large defects will induce heart failure and need surgical closure. Other defects may be operated on later if they fail to close spontaneously.

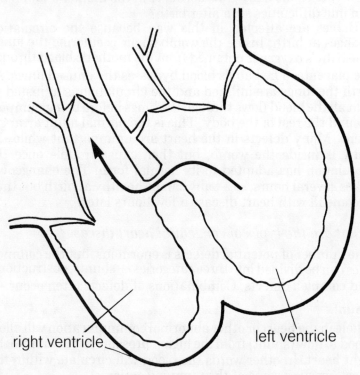

right ventricle

left ventricle

Figure 5.3. Ventricular septal defect

Patent ductus arteriosus (PDA)

The ductus arteriousus is a vessel which connects the pulmonary artery to the aorta so that the blood can bypass the lungs while the baby is inside the womb. After birth the vessel is no longer required and should close within a few days. Sometimes it does not, so blood in the aorta can\ shunt back into the pulmonary artery, reducing the pumping efficiency of the heart (Figure 5.4).

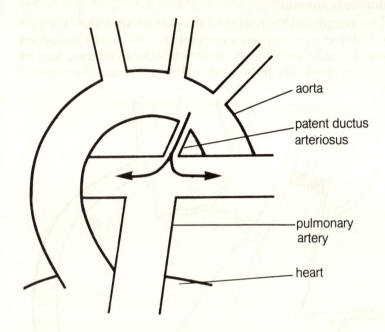

Figure 5.4. Patent ductus arteriosus

A patent ductus arteriosus is often a trivial problem with the murmur being heard at a routine examination. By today's standards, surgical closure is a simple operation and is readily carried out if necessary. In a few babies, particularly premature ones, the patent ductus can induce heart failure. An emergency operation may be needed to close it.

Obstructions

The normal blood flow within or out of the heart can be obstructed by congenitally stenosed valves or a narrowed aorta. The subject has already been mentioned earlier in this chapter. The pressure behind the obstruction rises, inducing enlargement (hypertrophy) of the relevant cardiac chamber. If the stress is excessive the muscle of that chamber may be permanently damaged.

Pulmonary stenosis

This congenital narrowing of the pulmonary valve is often a trivial defect of no consequence (Figure 5.5). In the few severe cases the right ventricle is under considerable stress and an operation to split the pulmonary valve (pulmonary valvotomy) will be needed.

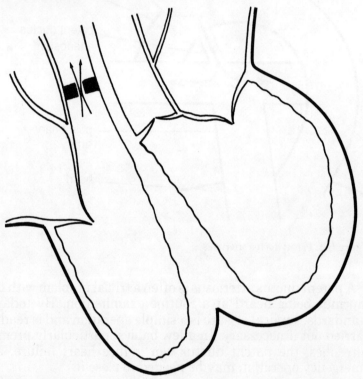

Figure 5.5. Pulmonary stenosis

Aortic stenosis

The narrowing can be at the valve, just below it, or just above it (Figure 5.6). Although many examples are trivial, doctors often keep the child under regular review as the narrowing may worsen. Surgery will often involve a complete valve replacement.

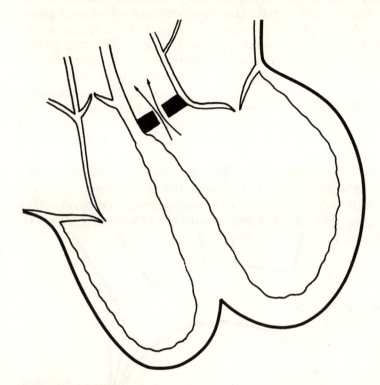

Figure 5.6. Aortic stenosis

Coarctation of the aorta

A coarctation is a narrowing of the aorta after it has given off the arteries to the head and arms (Figure 5.7). The strain on the left ventricle, trying to pump the blood through this resistance, can produce heart failure. A coarctation is also a rare cause of hypertension (p.86). The pressure in the upper half of the body rises in order to force the blood down to the lower half. A coarctation can be corrected at operation, though this does not always reverse long-standing hypertension.

Complex defects

Cyanosis is a feature of many of the more complex congenital heart defects. Venous, deoxygenated, blood has a bluey-purple tinge, while arterial blood normally contains more oxygen and is a much brighter red. The blood changes colour as it passes through the lungs and the oxygen is taken up. With many complex defects some of the blood bypasses the lungs. The arteries then contain deoxygenated blood which gives the skin, lips and tongue a bluey-purplish appearance. This is known as cyanosis and affected children are often called 'blue babies', though the term is an inadequate description of a subtle colour change. Peripheral cyanosis of the hands and feet is common if they become very cold, but heart defects produce central cyanosis — cyanosis involving the whole body.

Not only is the child's colour abnormal, but the organs may also have difficulty in obtaining sufficient oxygen. The body attempts to alleviate this by producing more red blood cells to carry oxygen. This reaction is not very helpful as it makes the

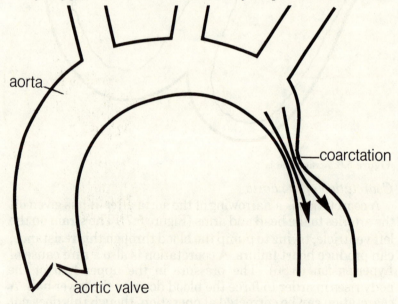

Figure 5.7. Coarctation of the aorta

blood thicker. The viscous blood is more difficult to pump around the body, placing an additional strain on the diseased heart. The blood may clot in inappropriate places. For several reasons the chronic cyanosis of some form of congenital heart disease is a debilitating condition.

Fallot's tetralogy

This combination of four abnormalities is the commonest cause of a cyanosed child after the first year of life. The defects are (Figure 5.8):

Pulmonary stenosis
Ventricular septal defects
Right ventricular hypertrophy
Abnormal position of the aorta.

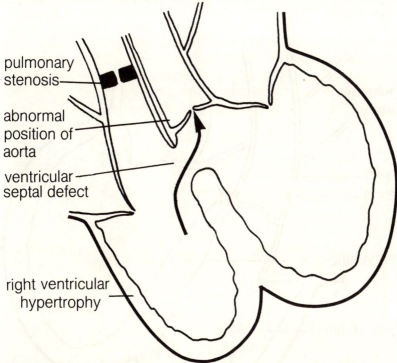

Figure 5.8. Fallot's tetralogy

The pulmonary stenosis obstructs the flow of deoxygenated blood which then crosses into the left heart through the ventricular septal defect, producing cyanosis when the blood is pumped around the body. Children with this condition often squat down during exercise to relieve their breathlessness. Fallot's tetralogy is amenable to surgery.

Transposition of the great vessels

In its simplest form the major vessels are transposed so that the right heart ejects blood into the aorta and the left heart into the pulmonary artery (Figure 5.9). If that was the only abnormality the baby could not survive more that a few minutes as the blood flow to the lungs would be entirely separate from the rest of the circulation. But a hole in the heart usually allows mixing of the blood. Deoxygenated blood can get into the arterial system, producing cyanosis. More complicated forms of transposition are also found.

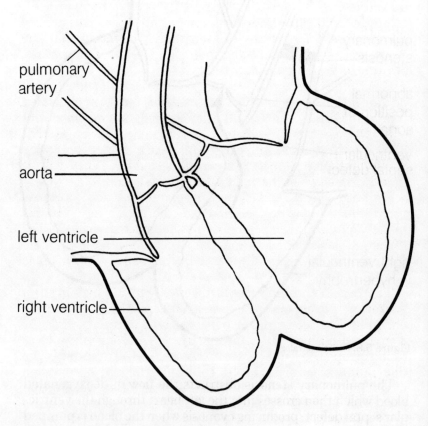

Figure 5.9. Transposition of the great vessels

A transposition can usually be dealt with surgically, though complex forms can provide a considerable challenge.

The eight conditions described above together represent over 90 per cent of congenital heart disease. Almost any cardiac structure can fail to develop correctly or even not appear at all, but fortunately most other abnormalities are rare.

How are congenital defects diagnosed?

Sometimes the findings on examination are specific. The diagnosis may be clear but the severity is often more difficult to judge at the bedside. With other problems, particularly more complex forms, the examination may reveal that the heart disease is present but not indicate the exact cause. Investigations are necessary.

Congenital heart disease may not be discovered until adolescence or even later. In the past this omission was often due to the absence of routine examinations in childhood, but this is rarely the case today. A commoner reason is that some of the features of congenital heart disease are quite subtle and easy to miss in a wriggling toddler. They will be detected later when the child is larger and calmer.

A chest X-ray and an electrocardiogram (p.23) may provide useful clues but rarely a complete diagnosis; for example, hypertrophy of a cardiac chamber may be detected. A chest X-ray to show the heart silhouette may help (p.22). Once again it is more likely to provide pieces of evidence rather than reveal the whole story.

The development of echocardiography (p.32) has been of enormous benefit in the assessment of heart disease in children. The technique is particularly good at showing the shape and position of the heart structures which is the basic problem in congenital heart disease. As it produces no discomfort, echocardiography can be performed on children at any age. The pictures obtained are very clear as the thin chest wall of children produces little obstruction to the beam of sound waves.

Cardiac catheterization (p.37) is still required in some children in spite of the success of echocardiography. Measurements of pressure or blood flow will indicate the severity of simple defects if surgery is being considered. More complex abnormalities need angiography to appreciate the anatomy and to plan the best treatment. A general anaesthetic will be used if necessary. Cardiac catheterization is being used less often, but it still has a major role when an operation is being contemplated.

What is the outlook for children with heart defects?

The term 'congenital heart disease' covers abnormalities ranging from trivial roughening of the surface of a valve to a gross deformity which is incompatible with life outside the womb. The outlook is very variable, depending on the underlying problem.

Fortunately many defects are unimportant and will remain so throughout life. A slight narrowing of the pulmonary valve or a small secundum atrial septal defect will not cause any trouble even if the patient lives to be a hundred years old; though detailed investigations may be needed to ensure that the defect really is trivial. Some abnormalities will correct themselves. Fortunately the commonest problem, a ventricular septal defect, will often close spontaneously in the first few years of life.

Some defects do not cause any symptoms initially but may do so later in life. One example is a moderate-sized septal defect. One result of the shunting through this type of defect is that the blood flow to the lungs may be increased by a factor of two, three or even more. The extra flow may eventually alter the structure of the lungs, increasing their resistance to the blood passing through. This will raise the pressure in the right side of the heart. In a severe case the shunt across the defect may be reversed, delivering unoxygenated blood to the arterial circulation (Figure 5.10). Cyanosis will occur. This is known as the Eisenmenger state after the man who first described it. Even if the shunt does not reverse, the increased lung resistance may produce symptoms later in life and it cannot be corrected at that stage. This is the main reason why surgical closure is often recommended for moderate-sized septal defects even when they are not creating symptoms.

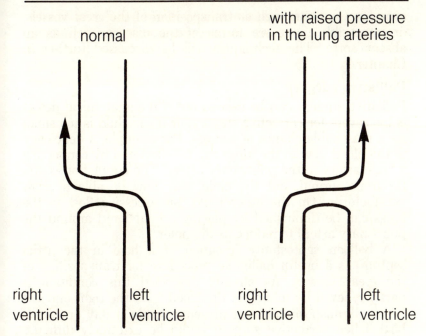

normal

with raised pressure
in the lung arteries

right
ventricle

left
ventricle

right
ventricle

left
ventricle

Figure 5.10. Ventricular septal defects

More severe abnormalities may be responsible for symptoms in childhood, particularly in the first few days and weeks after birth. Common symptoms in babies are cyanosis, breathlessness, feeding difficulties, and failure to thrive. Older children are more likely to have cyanosis, breathlessness, or tiredness. Once symptoms have occurred the outlook will depend on the chances of successful treatment, normally an operation. One exception is a patent ductus arteriosus which may produce heart failure soon after birth, but then close, perhaps with the help of drug therapy, and never produce any more trouble.

What is the treatment of congenital heart disease?

The definitive treatment of congenital heart disease is surgical correction. This can be relatively simple with a problem such as an atrial septal defect, more difficult with a complex condition such as transposition of the great vessels, or impossible in severe forms of the disease such as an absent aorta. The techniques will be discussed further in Chapter 7.

Palliative surgery

Palliative surgery can be carried out if the anatomical defect is too severe for corrective surgery, or if the child is too small for a reasonable chance of success. For example, a deficiency in the blood flow to the lungs can be alleviated by connecting a large artery to the pulmonary artery. The circulation is still far from normal, but the child may now be able to grow satisfactorily. On the other hand, an excessive flow to the lungs can be diminshed by placing a tight band around the pulmonary artery to reduce its diameter.

A balloon septostomy (creation of a hole in the atrial septum) is a useful palliative procedure for transposition of the great vessels. As already described this condition is partly relieved by mixing of the blood from the right and left hearts. Transposition often presents within a day or two of birth when corrective surgery would be extremely difficult. However, at cardiac catheterization a special catheter can be placed across the atrial septum in these newborn children. A balloon is blown up at the tip and the catheter is pulled back, creating a large hole in the septum. This alleviates the condition, allowing corrective surgery to be postponed until the child is bigger,

Drug therapy

Drug therapy has a fairly minor role in the treatment of congenital heart disease. Heart failure can be treated along the lines described on page 83. Paroxysms of extreme cyanosis in some complex lesions can be controlled by drug therapy.

Removal of venous blood

Regular venesections (removal of venous blood) may help some children with cyanosis that cannot be relieved by surgery. As we have seen, cyanosis produces an excess of red blood cells in an attempt to overcome the reduced oxygen concentration in the arterial blood. The increased blood viscosity worsens the load on the heart. Venesection will remove blood cells which. will be replaced by fluid from the rest of the body, reducing the thickness of blood. A venesection every few months may keep the blood viscosity at tolerable levels.

Heart muscle disease

Coronary artery disease and valve defects have been described earlier in this book. In addition a number of conditions are found where the main problem is disease of the heart muscle without any coronary artery disease. They can be divided into two groups depending on whether the cause of the muscle disorder is known. If it is, they are often referred to as 'specific muscle disease'; if not, 'cardiomyopathy' is a common description. Three types of cardiomyopathy have been described — hypertrophic, congestive, and restrictive.

Specific muscle disease

In general, the heart muscle is very resilient. Diseases which involve several organs often spare the heart. But a number of generalized diseases can affect the heart muscle, reducing its contractile power. Heart failure could follow if the problem is not resolved. Alcoholism is one example. Many alcoholics never develop any heart damage, but in some the heart muscle is severely affected. The dysfunction can be reversed by abstinence from alcohol. In some parts of the world a type of vitamin B deficiency (beri-beri) may involve the heart. By contrast a chronic excess of iron can result in heart disease. This cannot happen just by taking iron tablets, but children who have had a large number of blood transfusions, which contain iron, for certain forms of anaemia may be affected. Several other diseases which involve many organs can damage the heart, though fortunately none are common.

A rather different form of specific muscle disease is when excessive demands are placed on the heart. The heart has to work hard, even at rest, and its muscle is under considerable strain. The best example is an overactive thyroid gland (thyrotoxicosis). In this condition the thyroid gland drives the heart all the time; a cardiac output which would be appropriate when running for a bus is maintained continously. The ventricular muscle may not manage and heart failure can follow.

Hypertrophic cardiomyopathy

The main feature of hypertrophic cardiomyopathy is an abnormal thickening (hypertrophy) of the left ventricular muscle. In other patients the muscle can hypertrophy in response to a chronic strain such as high blood pressure, but this thickening has no known cause. One theory is that it is an abnormal reponse to catecholamines in the blood.

The thickened muscle can outstrip its blood supply, even though the coronary arteries are normal. Toxic chemicals may build up and produce pain. This pain has the same characteristics such as angina, except that it does not necessarily have the typical relationship to exercise. For this reason its cardiac origin may be missed initially. Another possible symptom is breathlessness. The thickened muscle bulges into the ventricular cavity. It is difficult to fill the ventricle properly so the volume of blood pumped is reduced. The resulting heart failure will be noticed as breathlessness. A third complication is an abnormal heart rhythm. The hyper-trophied muscle slows the spread of electricity with each heart beat (p.10). Not all the ventricular muscle is excited at the same time so the spread of electricity can become uncoordinated, producing abnormal rhythms.

The diagnosis may be suspected on examination. The thickened muscle can partly obstruct the outflow from the left ventricle, creating a murmur. The hypertrophy may be felt as a forceful beat on the outside of the chest wall. The electrocardiogram can document the hypertrophy, though it will not distinguish it from thickening due to other causes. The key to the diagnosis is the echocardiogram (p.32) where the thickened muscle is seen together with characteristic patterns of movement of the mitral and aortic valves.

Many examples of hypertrophic cardiomyopathy occur in isolation, but it can run in families. These familial cases are often minor, asymptomatic forms, picked up by echocardigraphy.

Most never cause any trouble, though a few may progress later. For this reason echocardiography is often performed on the children of patients with hypertrophic cardiomyopathy to pick up familial forms.

The treatment of hypertrophic cardiomyopathy has improved considerably in recent years. At one time the symptoms were difficult to control, but several drugs are now available. Propranolol (Inderal), a beta-blocking agent which is also used for angina, hypertension and abnormal rhythms, limits the muscle thickening and can be used long-term for pain or breathlessness. Verapamil (Cordilox), a calcium antagonist used for angina and abnormal rhythms, also seems to be useful though its role has not yet been fully evaluated. If an abnormal heart rhythm is the main problem, amiodarone (Cordarone X) is particularly effective. In severe cases, surgical resection of some of the thickened muscle may allow the ventricle to pump better but such an operation is rarely needed.

Congestive cardiomyopathy

In this heart muscle disease the muscle loses some of its contractile power; it goes 'flabby'. After a myocardial infarction some of the muscle is permanently damaged and no longer contracts; but that is a patchy phenomenon. With congestive cardiomyopathy all the muscle of the left ventricle is contracting poorly.

The cause is uncertain. One theory is that it is a response to an earlier virus infection. The heart can certainly be affected by viruses. The resulting inflammation of the heart, known as a myocarditis, can produce transient heart failure. But the inflammation burns itself out within a few days or weeks and the heart usually returns to normal. Detailed investigations of patients with congestive cardiomyopathy sometimes reveal evidence of previous virus infections and it may be that some viruses can produce a more chronic form of muscle damage.

Breathlessness and tiredness due to heart failure are the main symptoms. Pain is not a feature. The heart enlarges in an attempt to maintain its output and this can be seen on a chest X-ray. Sometimes it is difficult to distinguish congestive cardiomyopathy from other forms of heart failure and echocardiography or catheterization may be needed to clarify the cause.

Treatment involves controlling the heart failure as described earlier (p.82). Research is being carried out on methods of reversing the muscle damage, but there is no general agreement yet on the best way of achieving this.

Restrictive cardiomyopathy

This type of cardiomyopathy is rarer than the hypertrophic or congestive forms. Fibrosis occurs in the heart muscle, making it stiff. The muscle movement, which is essential for filling and emptying of the left ventricle, is then restricted. The cause is unknown, though the condition is associated with an increase in the numbers of some white blood cells known as eosinophils and it is assumed that they are involved in some way.

Breathlessness and tiredness secondary to heart failure are the main symptoms. Drug therapy is helpful, though surgical resection of the fibrous tissue is the best treatment if it is technically possible.

Pericarditis

The pericardium is a thin membrane which surrounds the heart, separating it from the lungs and other organs.

Acute pericarditis

The pericardium may become inflamed, particularly as the result of a virus infection. This is known as acute pericarditis. It can also be secondary to other problems, such as kidney failure or a myocardial infarction. Acute viral pericarditis is a benign illness, but it has to be distinguished from other more important forms of heart disease. Chest pain is the main symptom together with a raised temperature. The pain is sharper and more stabbing than true cardiac pain and there is no relationship to exercise. Pericardial pain is often relieved by sitting up, but is made worse by deep inspiration. Cardiac pain is unaffected by breathing. The diagnosis may be confirmed by hearing a typical scratchy sound with the stethoscope and by electrocardiographic changes.

Acute viral pericarditis is a self-limiting condition which resolves spontaneously within days or weeks, though it can be very painful. The main problem is the unnecessary anxiety it can generate in a young person whose heart is normal. The outlook for other forms of acute pericarditis depends on the underlying cause.

Pericardial effusion

Fluid trapped between the pericardium and the heart is known as a pericardial effusion. Acute pericarditis is a common cause, but it can also occur with some non-cardiac diseases, notably those of the kidney. A pericardial effusion rarely causes any symptoms but it will increase the size of the heart shadow on a chest X-ray. This has to be distinguished from other, more serious, causes of an enlarged heart shadow, such as heart failure secondary to coronary artery disease. In a few patients the volume of fluid is sufficiently large to raise the pressure inside the pericardial sac and restrict the filling of the heart. Symptoms of heart failure will then appear.

A pericardial effusion may be suspected on examination but an echocardiogram is very effective in demonstrating the excess fluid around the heart. In asymptomatic patients no treatment is required, though some of the fluid may be extracted through a needle for diagnostic purposes. In the few patients with symptoms drainage of the fluid will produce rapid relief. Repeated aspirations or surgical removal of the pericardium may be needed if the fluid re-accumulates.

Constrictive pericarditis

In this rare disease the pericardium becomes thick and fibrous over several years. Previous tuberculosis is one cause, but many cases do not seem to have a particular antecedent event. Like restrictive cardiomyopathy, constrictive pericarditis limits the normal filling of the heart. The cardiac outputs is diminished, producing heart failure. Surgical removal of the constricting pericardium is the best treatment but it can be difficult.

127

Pulmonary hypertension

Raised blood pressure in the arteries which supply the body is known as hypertension, or more accurately systemic hypertension. Pulmonary hypertension is an elevated pressure in the pulmonary artery which carries blood to the lungs. This increased pressure places a strain on the right ventricle which has thinner muscle than the left ventricle and is not designed to pump blood at a high pressure. The right ventricle will dilate and right heart failure (p.83) will follow. Some tricuspid incompetence secondary to the dilatation may worsen the failure. The increased pressure in the pulmonry artery may also produce incompetence of the pulmonary valve though this is never of any functional importance.

The pulmonary hypertension can be secondary to some lung diseases. The damage from severe chronic bronchitis or emphysema will increase the resistance to blood flow, elevating the pressure in the arteries proximal to the lungs. The right heart failure produced by the pulmonary hypertension secondary to these conditions is known as cor pulmonale. Another cause of pulmonary hypertension is blood clots. The clots (thrombi) in the leg veins can break free and travel to the lungs in the circulation. They are called pulmonary emboli. By obstructing the blood flow to the lungs, they can embarrass the circulation or damage part of these organs. If they recur frequently, pulmonary hypertension may follow.

Heart disease may produce pulmonary hypertension. We have already seen how the chronic increase in lung blood flow with certain congenital defects can elevate the pulmonary artery pressure. Mitral valve disease can also increase the pressure. Mitral stenosis or incompetence can 'dam up' the blood in the left atrium. In order to drive the blood through the lungs and into the left atrium, the pulmonary artery pressure has to rise a little. But sometimes this rise is excessive, creating pulmonary hypertension in addition to the mitral valve disease.

A few examples of pulmonary hypertension do not have any apparent cause. The patients are usually young to middle-aged women. The resistance of the blood vessels in the lungs increases for no good reason. This is known as primary pulmonary hypertension.

The best treatment is to correct the underlying cause of the pulmonary hypertension. For example, anticoagulant drugs (p.70) will prevent further emboli if this is the basic problem. If the causes cannot be resolved, treatment is difficult. Continuous inhalation of oxygen in severe chronic bronchitis improves lung blood flow and can reduce the pulmonary hypertension, though the chronic inhalation is very arduous. Unlike 'ordinary' hypertension, it is difficult to lower the pressure in the pulmonary artery by drug therapy. Some drugs can help but intensive monitoring may be needed to make sure that they are not doing more harm than good.

Dissection of the aorta

This rare, serious condition can occur in people with uncontrolled hypertension or with an abnormal aorta. The initial event is a break in the internal surface of the aorta. Blood at high, arterial pressure then pushes apart the layers of the aortic wall (Figure 5.11). This is known as a dissection. If it stops or ruptures back into the lumen of the aorta the consequences may not be severe. But it can burst outwards to produce a dangerous haemorrhage.

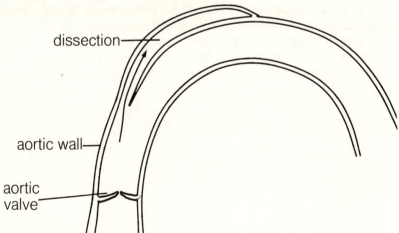

Figure 5.11. Dissection of the aorta

The main symptom is severe chest pain, often radiating through to the back. The dissection can spread backwards to involve the aortic valve and other cardiac structures. Immediate angiography (p.38) is required to confirm the diagnosis and find which part of the aorta is involved. The initial treatment is to lower the blood pressure by drugs to reduce the risk of further spread. Some dissections, especially those involving the aorta nearest the heart, need surgery to prevent increasing damage.

Tumours of the heart

Fortunately, heart tumours are very rare. They can originate in the heart (primary tumour) or they can be secondary to a malignant tumour (cancer) elsewhere in the body. The heart is less liable to develop cancer than almost any other organ.

The primary tumours are usually slow growing, non-malignant, tumours which do not spread outside the heart. But even a small tumour can cause trouble if it involves a valve or the electrical conducting system. One type of tumour, a myxoma, may shed bits into the circulation. These emboli can block arteries in a similar manner to the thrombotic emboli from the left atrium (p.103). A myxoma can be readily removed at operation.

Secondary tumours from cancer elsewhere in the body can occasionally affect the heart. The cells arrive in the blood stream or spread directly from the nearby lungs. On the rare occasions when the heart is involved, usually the tumours are already widespread. Treatment is directed at killing the malignant cells throughout the body by chemical means.

6

Abnormal rhythms and pacemakers

Abnormal heart rhythms can complicate many forms of heart disease and they can also appear in isolation. So it is convenient to describe them in a separate chapter. Abnormal rhythms are due to a malfunction of the electrical system of the heart which is often called the conducting system. The healthy conducting system has already been described in Chapter 2. For simplicity, its components can be summarized in a diagram (Figure 6.1). The electrical activity starts spontaneously in the sinus node and then spreads across the atria to initiate atrial contraction. The normal rhythm is called sinus rhythm. The activity passes slowly through the atrioventricular node then quickly down the bundle of His to activate the ventricles. The delay in the atrioventricular node is essential for the correct sequence of atrial contraction followed by ventricular contraction about a fifth of a second later.

If the normal system fails, stand-by mechanisms ensure that the heart continues beating, though perhaps not at the correct rate. These reserve mechanisms involve 'potential pacemaker' cells. During normal sinus rhythm the potential pacemaker cells are excited by the spread of electricity before they have time to initiate any activity themselves. But if the electricity does not arrive, they will 'fire off' spontaneously, starting a wave of electricity which can spread to other parts of the heart if necessary. The potential pacemaker cells are a blessing when they maintain the heart rhythm, but they can be a nuisance if they start firing at a fast rate, producing an abnormal rhythm. They are found in all parts of the heart.

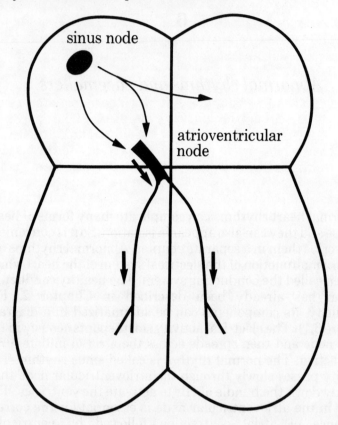

Figure 6.1. The conducting system

The conducting system is designed to trigger a heart beat about once a second for a century or more if necessary. Contrary to a popular belief, the heart beat is not always regular in healthy people. In the young the rate varies with breathing; the heart speeds up on breathing in and slows down on breathing out. This normal phenomenon is known as a sinus arrhythmia. Many people have extra beats. These early contractions, also known as premature or ectopic beats, are due to the ventricles, or the conducting system above the ventricles firing off spontaneously before the normal electrical activity arrives from the sinus node. They may be called ventricular or supraventricular ectopic beats. Occasional early beats are so common that they can hardly be regarded as abnormal. They rarely produce symptoms and the person is usually unaware of their existence.

The heart rate of a healthy person *at rest* is usually between 55 and 110 beats per minute. But it can be outside this range under certain circumstances. For example, the heart may slow below 55 per minute during sleep. A highly trained athlete will often have a slow pulse at rest which returns to the normal range during exertion. During strenuous exercise most people can have a rate of up to 150-200 per minute. Anxiety or pain can produce a similar increase. Conversely, an abnormal rhythm is not always outside the range of 55-110 beats per minute. But an abnormal rhythm within these values is unlikely to produce any serious effects.

Abnormal heart rhythms can either be too fast or too slow. They are known as tachycardias or bradycardias respectively. In a tachycardia a fast rhythm has suppressed the slower sinus rhythm. A bradycardia occurs when the conducting system is not initiating or conducting the normal electrical impulse and a potential pacemaker has taken over. Some patients have a mixture, with periods of slow rhythm interspersed with rapid beating.

Fast rhythms

Fast rhythms (tachycardias) can be divided into two groups — those arising from abnormally fast beating of the ventricles (ventricular tachycardia) and those created by fast beating atria or the atrioventricular node (supraventricular tachycardia). Ventricular tachycardias are faster and so tend to produce more severe symptoms than supraventricular tachycardias.

The supraventricular arrhythmias can take three different forms. *Atrial fibrillation* has already been mentioned in the context of mitral valve disease, but it often occurs under other circumstances. With this rhythm the electrical activity of the atria becomes uncoordinated, so that at any one moment some of the atrial muscle is contracting and some relaxing. The end result is that the electrical impulse passes through the atrioventricular node to the ventricles in an erractic fashion, producing an irregular heart beat. If the atrial activity becomes rather more coordinated, *atrial flutter* may be the result. The atrial contraction is still abnormal but regular activity is seen on the electrocardiogram. In an *atrial tachycardia* the atria are being driven at a fast rate but the pattern of atrial excitation is relatively normal.

A rapid heart beat may be due to sinus tachycardia. This is the normal speeding up of the heart in response to exertion, pain, or emotion. It can be quite fast, but it is not an abnormal rhythm. Unfortunately a few people worry that it represents heart disease which in turn makes the rate even faster. Occasionally, detailed investigations are needed to reassure the person that the heart is normal. The relief of anxiety will break the circle of events. In this book tachycardia will refer to abnormal fast rhythms, not to sinus tachycardia which is the normal rhythm at an increased rate.

What causes tachycardias?

One cause is a small part of the heart ('focus') acting as an abnormal pacemaker. Then the rapid electrical activity will spread to the rest of the atria or ventricles. This abnormal focus may occur in association with coronary artery disease, valvular heart disease, congenital defects, cardiomyopathies, or other forms of heart disease. It can also be produced in normal hearts by an excessive dose of some drugs or abnormalities in the minerals in the blood. A few patients develop a focus without any demonstrable problem.

Another way to generate an abnormal tachycardia is a 'circus movement'. An essential property of atrial and ventricular muscle is that once it has already been electrically excited it is unresponsive to further stimulation for about a quarter of a second. This means that normally the electricity can only move down the heart; backwards spread is blocked by unresponsive muscle. But if the electricity is delayed by abnormal muscle which can only conduct slowly, the cells higher up in the heart may have had time to recover and the electricity can travel backwards (Figure 6.2). It can then come down through healthy muscle and go back to excite the healthy muscle again. A self-perpetuating circus movement has been established.

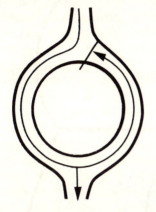 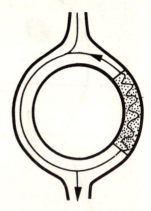

Figure 6.2. Principle of circus movement tachycardias

The circus will drive the rest of the atria or ventricles at the faster rate. As with an abnormal focus, the slow-conducting muscle of a circus can be produced by a wide variety of heart diseases or it may occur in the absence of any other demonstrable problem.

A specific cause of circus movement tachycardias is the Wolff-Parkinson-White syndrome (WPW). In this condition, which is named after the three doctors who first described it, the patient has an extra communication between the atria and ventricles. In most people the atrioventricular node and the bundle of His represent the only electrical link between the two types of chambers. But in the Wolff-Parkinson-White syndrome, a minor congenital abnormality produces an extra bridge of muscle (bundle of Kent), providing another electrical link (See Figure 6.3). The syndrome usually does not create symptoms and is often seen as an incidental finding in an electrocardiogram done for another purpose. But it can be responsible for circus movement tachycardias. The electricity can travel down the bridge of muscle and then back up to the bundle of His and the atrioventricular node to produce the necessary circular motion. Or it can spread down the bundle of His and back up to the muscle bridge.

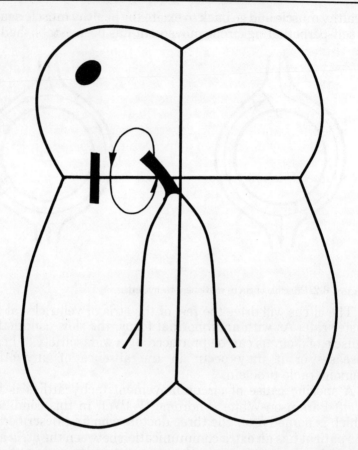

Figure 6.3. Wolff-Parkinson-White syndrome producing circus movement tachycardia

What are the symptoms of a tachycardia?

The nature and severity of any symptoms are variable, depending on the speed of the tachycardia and the presence of any other cardiac or non-cardiac disease. A tachycardia which would hardly be noticed in a healthy young person, can create severe trouble in an old patient with chronic heart failure or a partially obstructed blood flow to the brain. Many tachycardias never produce symptoms and are only discovered by chance.

The most obvious symptoms of a tachycardia is an awareness of the rapid heart beat. This may be described as 'palpitations' or a 'fluttering in the chest'. The patient may notice the change from a regular to an irregular rhythm rather than an alteration in the rate. But a feeling of palpitations is not diagnostic of an abnormal heart rhythm. Many people are aware of a normal rhythm at times, particularly when they are still in bed at night. Palpitations are often due to a normal heart beat which in turn is speeded up by unnecessary worry that the palpitations are due to heart disease. Abnormal tachycardias tend to occur at any time of the day, and they start and stop suddenly. Awareness of a normal heart beat often manifests itself at certain times of the day and usually fades away gradually. But investigations may be needed to distinguish these two conditions.

The symptoms of a tachycardia may be less precise. The pumping efficiency of the heart is reduced by the excess rate so the symptoms can be those of a low cardiac output — tiredness, lack of energy. Patients may feel unwell, but be unable to provide a more accurate description. A temporary reduction in the blood flow to the brain may produce a transitory unsteadiness or even loss of consciousness, though this latter symptom is unusual.

Tachycardias may be paroxysmal, in which case the symptoms will be intermittent, or persistent when the symptoms may continue for a long period. In general symptoms are worst at the onset of a tachycardia; the heart can partly adjust to the fast rate.

How are tachycardias diagnosed?

The existence of a tachycardia can be suspected from the story or the examination, but an electrocardiogram is normally required for confirmation. On examination a persistent tachycardia will appear as an inappropriately fast pulse rate. An electrocardiogram (p.23) will be used to confirm that an abnormal tachycardia is present and to indicate its type. A paroxysmal tachycardia can be more difficult to demonstrate. A patient may describe palpitations or other symptoms at times during the day but nothing may be felt when the doctor is present and examination only reveals normal rhythm. Ambulatory rhythm. Ambulatory monitoring of the electrocardiogram (p.30) may be able to document an occasional tachycardia. Some hospitals have special instruments that transmit the electrocardiogram down the telephone. A patient can take such an instrument home and when tachycardia starts he 'phones in' the abnormal heart rhythm for analysis.

Are tachycardias serious?

Supraventricular tachycardias are usually not dangerous, though they can generate severe symptoms in a few patients. If other forms of heart disease are present, the onset of a supraventricular tachycardia may produce a temporary deterioration in cardiac function. Heart failure may worsen or angina could be induced. Sometimes the tachycardia can be disabling itself, particularly in older patients. But supraventricular tachycardias are not dangerous because the atrioventricular node protects the ventricles. However fast the atria are beating, the ventricles cannot be driven above the maximum rate that the node can conduct the electricity — normally less than 200 times a minute. The ventricles can still fill and empty at this speed so the circulatory disturbance is not profound. The main exception is an occasional patient with the Wolff-Parkinson-White syndrome (p.135). The muscle bridge bypasses the atrioventricular node and may allow the ventricles to be driven at the same rapid rate as the atria. Drugs will be required to limit the speed of conduction through the muscle bridge.

Ventricular tachycardias may be more serious. In this rhythm the rapid beating is triggered by the ventricles, so the atrioventricular node has no protective effect. The rate can be so rapid that the ventricles can no longer fill and empty satisfactorily, and the cardiac output is drastically reduced. This may be dangerous if the tachycardia is not treated promptly.

What causes dropped beats?

A feeling that the heart misses a beat is quite a common sensation. A heart beat is not really absent; a contraction has come early, which leaves a longer period before the next one. This short pause produces the 'dropped beat' sensation. The early beats are known as premature or ectopic beats and they have already been mentioned as a cause of an irregular heart beat in healthy people. They arise spontaneously in the ventricles (ventricular ectopic beats) or in the conducting system above the ventricles (supraventricular ectopic beats).

Are dropped beats important?

Many dropped beats occur in the absence of heart disease. Under these circumstances they are unimportant apart from being a mild nuisance if they are felt frequently. If necessary drug therapy will eliminate them, though reassurance may be all that is necessary.

Sometimes the ectopic beats are associated with heart abnormalities such as coronary artery disease. But the subject will nearly always have other symptoms of heart disease before the dropped beats are noticed. Ectopic beats as the first indication of heart trouble is very rare. Occasionally, ventricular ectopic beats occcurring in conjunction with some forms of heart disease can progress to ventricular tachycardia or other rhythm abnormalities. So doctors may recommend drugs to control the ectopic beats even if they have not produced any significant symptoms. This will prevent the occurrence of a potentially serious ventricular rhythm disturbance.

What is the treatment of tachycardias?

In general, tachycardias can be treated in three ways:

Do nothing
Drugs
Electricity.

Many tachycardias do not require any treatment. This is particularly true with brief paroxysms of a supraventricular tachycardia. The symptoms may be so brief and intermittent that chronic daily drug therapy would not be worthwhile. This may also be true of some persistent supraventricular tachycardias, such as slow atrial fibrillation, when the rate is similar to that of a normal rhythm. The more serious ventricular tachycardias will usually require some form of treatment.

Drug therapy may be used to terminate a tachycardia, to

control the ventricular rate with a chronic supraventricular tachycardia, or to prevent a tachycardia recurring. A variety of drugs are used, reflecting the fact that none of the available agents is ideal. It can be difficult to predict which drug will be the most effective for a particular patient and some 'trial and error' may be needed to find the best agent. Some of the commoner drugs will be described below.

Supraventricular tachycardias

Digoxin (Lanoxin)

This drug is often effective in controlling the ventricular rate of a supraventricular tachycardia. It may be able to terminate such a tachycardia, and it can be given long-term to reduce the risk of a recurrence. Digoxin is also used for treatment of heart failure, so a combination of the two conditions is a good indication for the drug. As mentioned in Chapter 3, its main disadvantage is that the toxic dose is not much greater than the therapeutic dose; so careful adjustment of the number of tablets may be needed.

Verapamil (Cordilox)

An intravenous injection of this drug may terminate a supraventricular tachycardia. The tablets are useful in controlling the ventricular rate or in preventing a reccurrence. The drug is also used in the treatment of angina.

Beta blockers

These drugs have already been mentioned for the treatment of angina and hypertension. They are also useful in terminating and preventing some supraventricular tachycardias. One of their advantages is that they may control both an abnormal tachycardia and a rapid, normal heart rhythm secondary to anxiety. So they can be used when it is uncertain which of these conditions is the cause of occasional palpitations.

Amiodarone (Cordarone X)

This is a new agent which is very effective with most supraventricular tachycardias. But its side-effects mean that it is rarely used as the first-choice drug. The commonest side-effect is a skin rash in response to sunlight. The drug is also deposited in small quantities in the front of the eye. This rarely seems to affect vision, but if it does, stopping the drug will allow the deposits to disperse.

Ventricular tachycardias

Lignocaine (Xylocard)

Ventricuar tachycardias are often treated in hospital with intravenous lignocaine; the drug is not effective by mouth. Lignocaine is used to terminate the tachycardias and also to prevent them, particularly in the first few hours after a myocardial infarction when ventricular arrhythmias are common (p.65).

Disopyramide (Rythmodan)

This drug is very useful in preventing ventricular tachy-cardias. An intravenous form is also available for terminating them. Some patients with difficulty in passing urine or excessive pressure inside the eyes (glaucoma) may find these conditions worsened by disopyramide.

Mexiletine (Mexetil), tocainide (Tonocard), procainamide (Pronestyl)

These agents have rather similar effects and can be given by injection to terminate a tachycardia or by mouth to prevent it. Their actions are not identical and if one does not work, another may be tried. They may produce nausea and vomiting in a few patients.

Amiodarone and the beta-blocking agents may also be helpful for controlling ventricular tachycardias. Quinidine is another drug employed for this purpose in some countries, but it is rarely used in Britain.

What is the electrical treatment of tachycardias?

As we have seen, many tachycardias are due to a 'circus movement' with the electrical activity going round and round inside the heart. If the circus movement is interrupted, the tachycardia will be terminated. This can be done by delivering a brief, powerful, electric shock through the heart. All the electrical activity of the heart is abolished for a fraction of a second by the shock, terminating the continuous circus movement. This shock technique, known as cardioversion, may also terminate atrial fibrillation by stopping the abnormal atrial activity and allowing a normal rhythm to re-emerge.

Cardioversion can be used for both supraventricular and ventricular tachycardias. The patient is first given a general anaesthetic, as the shock would be painful. Two metal paddles are applied to either side of the chest and the brief burst of current passes between them. The patient wakes up a few minutes later. The only after-effect is that the paddles sometimes leave a red ring on the skin; this disappears within a few days. One potential risk of cardioversion in patients with long-standing atrial fibrillation is that a blood clot might be released from the left atrium to form an embolus (p.103) as the rhythm is returned to normal. These patients are often anticoagulated (p.104) for a few weeks prior to the cardioversion to prevent this complication. Cardioversion can only be done in hospital by doctors with the necessary experience. But it has the big advantage of an immediate effect and avoidance of some drug side-effects.

More subtle electrical ways of terminating a tachycardia are being developed, though their application is limited at present. As described later in this chapter, pacemakers are normally used to control slow heart rhythms. But special models are being made to stimulate the heart in such a way that the tachycardia is stopped. The stimulation causes no discomfort so, unlike a cardioversion, this method can be used repeatedly. The technique has only recently been introduced and its place in therapy is not yet established.

Do tachycardias go away?

Not suprisingly, this depends on the circumstances. Tachycardias which occur in the first few hours after a myocardial infarction will often disappear once the acute event is over. Similarly an abnormal rhythm secondary to an overdosage of drugs or a deficiency of certain minerals in the blood will resolve when the body returns to normal. But many tachycardias are due to chronic forms of heart disease without any immediate precipitating factor. In these patients the risk of a recurrence will persist as long as the heart disease is present, which may be for many years. If the tachycardia is potentially serious, long-term preventative drug therapy will be required.

Slow rhythms

As we have already seen, a slow heart is not necessarily abnormal. A rate of 40-55 beats per minute is not uncommon in some young people while asleep or in highly trained athletes while awake. But abnormal slow rhythms (bradycardias) are also fairly common. The two main types are heart block and the sick sinus syndrome.

Heart block is due to delayed or blocked electrical conduction in the atrioventricular node or the conducting system below the node (Figure 6.4). In other words conduction from the atria to the ventricles is affected. It appears in three forms:

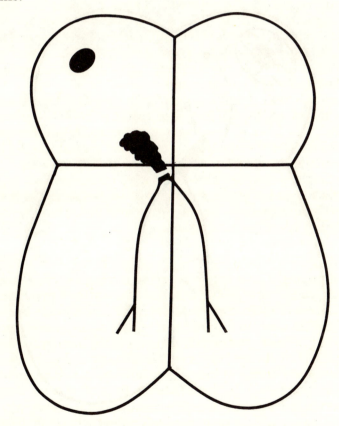

Figure 6.4. Complete heart block

143

1) First degree heart block. The electrocardiogram shows delayed conduction; but the heart rate is normal and no symptoms are produced.

2) Second degree heart block. Conduction from the atria to the ventricles is intermittent, so some electrical impulses get through and some do not. The heart will slow and become irregular but the change is rarely sufficient to create any symptoms.

3) Third degree heart block. None of the electrical activity of the atria is transmitted to the ventricles. It is also called complete heart block. The ventricles beat at their own slow rate and symptoms are fairly common.

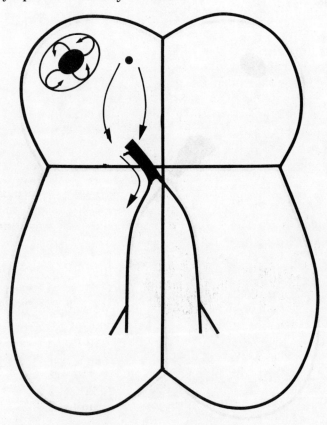

Figure 6.5. Sick sinus syndrome

The sick sinus syndrome is produced by a defect in the impulse formation at the sinus node and surrounding atrium (Figure 6.5) Unlike heart block when the atria continue beating normally, both the atria and the ventricles are slowed in the sick sinus syndrome. Sinus node disease and sinoatrial disease are alternative descriptions. Supraventricular tachycardias may also be found in the sick sinus syndrome.

What causes bradycardias?

The bradycardias of both heart block and the sick sinus syndrome can be induced by other types of heart disease, such as coronary artery disease. A short period of complete heart block is fairly common after a myocardial infarction. But the slow rhythms occur more frequently in the absence of other heart problems. In these patients, microscopic examination of the heart shows fibrosis of the conducting system; but the cause of the fibrosis is uncertain. Any sudden cardiac event, such as an unexpected faintness due to complete heart block, is popularly attributed to a heart attack; but in reality few of these arrhythmias are due to any form of coronary artery disease.

Whatever the cause of the fibrosis, complete heart block and the sick sinus syndrome are commonest in the elderly. Over the age of 80 years, about one person in 200 has a complete heart block which makes it a common disease. But bradycardias can be found at any age. Complete heart block can be a congenital defect, appearing at birth.

What are the symptoms of bradycardia?

The symptoms are characteristically variable and usually consist of some or all of tiredness, unsteadiness, faintness, and loss of consciousness. They are produced by a reduced blood supply to other organs, particularly the brain. The brain is dependent on a continuous blood supply. If it is interrupted, brain function will be interfered with. A severe bradycardia for only a few seconds is sufficient to make the patient feel unsteady. A few seconds more and temporary unconsciousness may follow. The degree of symptoms partly depends on the severity of the bradycardia and partly on the state of health of the brain and its blood vessels. An older person with narrowed arteries to the brain will be less able to tolerate a bradycardia than a young person. Similarly, symptoms will be worse if the bradycardia starts when the patient is standing up and the blood can drain away from the brain. For the same reason, a few patients have their worse symptoms when they get out of bed in the mornings.

Complete loss of consciousness secondary to a severe brady-cardia is known as a Stokes-Adams attack after the two Irish doctors who first described the condition. During an attack the patient will fall down, which minimizes the effects of the slow heart. Blood flow to the brain will improve in a horizontal patient. The symptoms of a Stokes-Adams attack are severe but brief, often only lasting for a few seconds. This can help in the diagnosis; loss of consciousness due to other causes usually persists far longer.

But the symptoms of a bradycardia are frequently more subtle. A persistent mild slowing of the heart can produce a non-specific feeling of tiredness. An episodic bradycardia may just create a transient unsteadiness for a fraction of a second. At times it is remarkable how a fairly severe bradycardia can produce no symptoms in an otherwise healthy patient.

How are bradycardias diagnosed?

Like tachycardias, the symptoms can be suggestive but every effort is made to obtain electrocardiographic confirmation. The bradycardia may be sufficiently persistent to be caught on an ordinary electrocardiogram. Intermittent slowing of the heart may be revealed by 24 hours of ambulatory monitoring (p.30).

Are bradycardias serious?

The slowing of the heart in the sick sinus syndrome is a nuisance, but it does not seem to be dangerous. As described earlier in this chapter, the heart has a number of 'potential-pacemaker' cells which will eventually drive the atria and ventricles if the sinus node is no longer functioning. The symptoms can be severe and may include injuries from falling to the ground, but the sick sinus syndrome is not otherwise dangerous.

The same potential-pacemaker cells in the ventricles will limit the duration of symptoms with complete heart block. But the conducting system is interrupted lower down in the heart; leaving fewer potential-pacemaker cells to take over. These cells are also less reliable than those in the atria. So a Stokes-Adams attack secondary to complete heart block can ooccasionally be dangerous. Most attacks do not result in any permanent harm, but the risk is there.

Are first and second degree heart block important?

At the most second degree heart block only produces minor symptoms and first degree produces none at all. But a patient can have first or second degree block most of the time with occasional episodes of complete heart block creating the symptoms, such as intermittent dizziness. So these lesser degrees of block have to be carefully evaluated.

How are bradycardias treated?

Like tachycardias, the options for bradycardias are to do nothing, to use drugs, or to institute electrical methods. An asymptomatic slowing of the heart in the sick sinus syndrome does not require any therapy. A similar reduction in the rate due to acquired complete heart block may need treatment to prevent trouble later. Congenital complete heart block is a more benign condition and is not treated until symptoms appear.

Drugs can help in the immediate relief of a bradycardia, but they are not very effective for long-term therapy. A sudden slowing can often be alleviated by drugs like atropine or isoprenaline given into the veins. A long-acting oral preparation of isoprenaline (Saventrine) is available for chronic use, but it is not always effective in maintaining a satisfactory ventricular rate without side-effects.

The mainstay of the control of bradycardias is electrical therapy in the form of temporary or permanent pacing. This will be described in the next section of this chapter.

Do bradycardias go away?

Some bradycardias, particularly those seen immediately after a myocardial infarction, are temporary and rarely recur. But many are not secondary to an acute event and they will tend to persist or

147

at least reappear intermittently. However, the interval between attacks may last for months or even years.

Pacemakers

Reliable cardiac pacing has been one of the major medical advances of the last 20 years. Modern pacemakers are very dependable and effective in the control of all types of bradycardias.

How do pacemakers work?

The basic cause of a bradycardia is that the ventricles are not stimulated by the heart's own electrical system at a sufficiently fast rate. A pacemaker will artificially stimulate the heart, producing contractions of both right and left ventricles at a suitable rate.

Fortunately only a small electrical current is required. Once a minute portion of the muscle has been excited, a wave of electricity is generated by the muscle cells and spreads across the ventricles. A typical pacemaker stimulus would be 5 thousandths of a Volt for half a thousandth of a second. The energy contained in such a brief stimulation is minute, enabling a battery under the skin to be used for permanent pacemakers.

What are the types of pacemakers and how are they inserted?

Pacemakers are either temporary (in place for a maximum of a few weeks) or permanent (designed to work for many years). They both share the same principle of delivering an electrical impulse to the ventricles, but the batteries and wires are different.

Temporary pacemakers

Temporary pacemakers are used to treat bradycardias which are likely to resolve spontaneously without risk of recurrence, or to control the ventricular rate in an emergency prior to the insertion of a permanent pacemaker. The temporary pacing 'wire' is placed in a large vein with the help of a local anaesthetic. The two common methods are a direct puncture of the vein running up from the arm (subclavain vein) in front of the shoulder, or a small incision to expose a vein at the elbow. Either side of the body may be used. With the help of an X-ray screen, the 'wire' is passed through to the heart and lodged at the end of the right ventricle (Figure 6.6). The muscle squeezes down on the tip of the 'wire' with each contraction holding it in place.

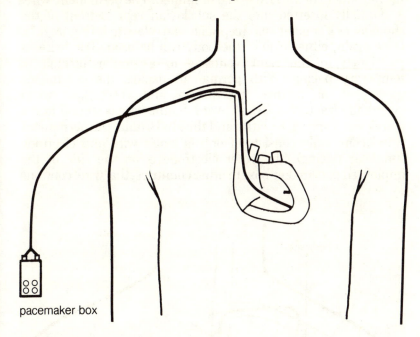

pacemaker box

Figure 6.6. Temporary pacing

The temporary 'wire' normally contains two separate insulated wires, wrapped in the same nonstick coating. One wire is connected to an electrode at the end of the 'wire' and the other to an electrode a centimetre or so further back. The ends of the wires outside the body are connected to a pacemaker box and brief bursts of current are passed between the electrodes to stimulate the heart. The 'threshold' is the minimum voltage that will excite the ventricles at any one time. The threshold rises in the first few days after insertion, so the initial threshold has to be low. The doctor may try different positions in the right ventricle to get a satisfactory low threshold. Once a good position has been found, the wire is fixed to the skin with a stitch and a dressing placed on top. The pacemaker box is left beside the bed or fixed to the patient's arm.

Permanent pacemakers

For a permanent pacemaker, veins at the elbow are not used as the movement of the arm would be limited. The permanent 'wire' is normally inserted into the subclavian vein in front of the shoulder or a smaller vein (cephalic vein) close to it (Figure 6.7). Once again, either side of the body can be used. The 'wire' is positioned in the right ventricle in a similar fashion to temporary pacing. With permanent pacing, the continuous movement of cardiac contraction and relaxation would eventually fracture a straight wire. So the wire is wound into a spiral, like a spring, to withstand this. In Britain, the permanent 'wire' commonly consists of only a single wire and electrode (unipolar pacing); the other electrode is on the side of the implanted pacemaker box. In other countries, the 'wire' contains

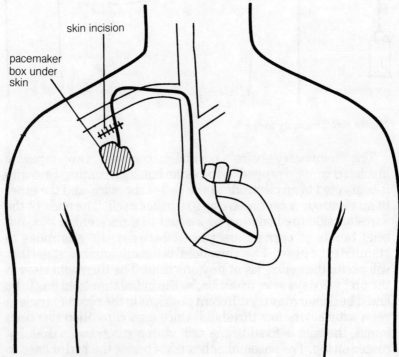

Figure 6.7. Permanent pacing

two wires and electrodes as in temporary pacing (bipolar pacing).

The permanent 'wire' is connected to the pacemaker box which is nowadays not much bigger than a thin matchbox. In the past they were much larger. The pacemaker box contains the batteries and electronics. It is inserted under the skin on the front of the chest wall. At the end of the procedure only the sutured wound and a slight bulge from the pacemaker box are visible. The pacemaker is checked a few days later and if there are no problems the patient can often go home within a few days of insertion.

How is a pacing 'wire' held in place permanently?

With the conventional technique, the tip of the 'wire' cannot be sewn on to the ventricular muscle in the manner of a surgical operation. Sometimes it does become displaced and will have to be repositioned. But this is not common. With correct placement. the ventricular muscle will tend to squeeze down on the 'wire', holding it firmly. The 'wires' are often made with knobs, flanges or screw-in devices at the tip which 'catch' on the muscular projections. But such devices are only needed temporarily. The natural defences of the body set up a fibrous reaction around the tip of the 'wire'. The fibres grow over the tip , binding it tightly to the muscle. Once the pacing 'wire' has been in position for a few weeks it cannot be displaced by the movement of the heart. Indeed, it can be difficult to remove it if this is required for some reason.

Who needs a pacemaker?

In general, a pacemaker is needed to control symptoms secondary to a slow heart rate. A few patients without symptoms also require a pacemaker to prevent a dangerous deterioration of their bradycardia.

The subject has been discussed earlier in this chapter. Specially designed pacemakers are sometimes used to interrupt tachycardias, but they do not yet have a general application. Ordinary pacemakers are only capable of speeding up the heart, not slowing it down. However, by maintaining a satisfactory rate they sometimes allow the dose of antitachycardia drugs to be increased to an effective level.

What symptoms will be helped by a pacemaker?

A pacemaker will only relieve symptoms secondary to a slow heart, such as loss of consciousness or dizziness. Symptoms which are primarily due to heart failure (breathlessness, tiredness) are sometimes helped by speeding up the heart, but often they are left unchanged. Angina is rarely improved by pacing.

Can children have a permanent pacemaker?

Yes, but there are difficulties. One is that the 'wire' does not grow with the child, so it may have to be changed as the child gets larger. Another is that the pacemaker box is relatively large in a baby or a toddler; it may be difficult to find a satisfactory place to implant it. Fortunately, few children need pacing.

What is a 'demand pacemaker'?

The earliest pacemakers paced continuously regardless of the underlying cardiac rhythm. But many bradycardias are only present intermittently and the normal rhythm often returned to compete with the paced rhythm. Almost all temporary and permanent pacemakers are now 'on demand'. The pacing electrodes are used to sense the natural heart beat and if the spontaneous ventricular rate slips below the rate for pacing, the pacemaker switches on. Once the pacemaker is on,the slower, natural rhythm is suppresed. But if the spontaneous rhythm becomes faster than the paced rhythm, the pacemaker switches off again.

What is a 'programmable pacemaker'?

Ordinary permanent pacemakers have a preset voltage and pacing rate. These values and other parameters connected with pacemaker function cannnot be altered during the lifetime of the pacemaker box. With a programmable pacemaker box, one or more of these parameters can be altered while the box is implanted. A programming device is placed on the skin over the box and an electromagnetic current is used to change the parameters. Programmable pacemakers are also demand pacemakers. They are used when an alteration in pacing function could be needed in the future. With an ordinary pace-maker, the box would have to be changed. With a programmable unit, the alterations can be done through the skin in a few seconds.

How long do the batteries last?

Permanent pacemakers have special lithium batteries with a remarkably long life. The duration of battery function depends on a number of variables such as its size and the task it is expected to perform. The batteries of most of today's pacemakers should last for at least 6 years and it is hoped that some will last for over 10 years. Older batteries had a shorter working life.

Replacement of a run-down battery is a simple operation. Under a general or local anaesthetic the old pacemaker box is removed and replaced with a new one. The 'wire' is tested and left undisturbed if it is working satisfactorily.

How long does the 'wire' last?

Ideally, a permanent 'wire' will last for the rest of the patient's life. But, as with any mechanical structure, faults do occur. If you consider that the 'wire' is bathed in the body fluids which have the corrosive properties of sea water and that it is bent and unbent seventy times a minute for years on end, its toughness becomes apparent. In the past 'wires' could be very unreliable. But most of the patients now receiving permanent pacemakers will never need another 'wire'.

How are permanent pacemakers checked?

There are two aspects to pacemaker function. Is the pacemaker generating a satisfactory stimulus? Is the stimulus triggering the ventricles? A satisfactory stimulus will achieve little if the 'wire' has moved and the electrode is no longer in contact with the muscle. An electrocardiogram (p.23) will reveal whether the ventricles are being driven by the pacemaker.

The commonest cause of an unsatisfactory stimulus is a run-down battery. The state of the battery in a pacemaker can be determined by measuring the pacing rate and the duration of the stimulus. Modern pacemakers are designed so that these values change in a predetermined manner as the batteries run down. Battery depletion can therefore be anticipated and the pacemaker box changed before pacing is lost. The necessary measurements can be done in a pacemaker clinic with a small instrument held on to the body surface. The pacing stimulus is detectable all over the upper half of the body. The checks are usually performed every 6-12 months.

If the heart has returned to a normal rate when the patient attends the clinic, the demand pacemaker will be switched off. In this state the stimulus cannot be analysed. The pacemaker can be temporarily switched on by a magnet placed over the box. The stimulus can then be checked.

Is a paced rhythm a normal rhythm?

No. It is close to a normal rhythm but there are differences. A normal heart speeds up with exercise but a paced rhythm is at a fixed rate. But the paced heart adapts in other ways (p.11) to increase its output during exercise. The fixed rate would be a disadvantage to a 4-minute miler, but in ordinary patients it produces no detectable disadvantage.

With a paced rhythm, the ventricles are the first part of the heart to be excited. In complete heart block the atria will beat independently at their own rate. In patients with the sick sinus syndrome the electrical activity will spread back up to the atria resulting in atrial activation *after* ventricular activation. With both conditions the correct timing of atrial contraction will be lost. Ventricular filling will be inhibited by a tendency for the tricuspid and mitral valves to close just as the atria are trying to push blood into the ventricles. The incorrect timing produces no ill effects in most patients, but a few with widespread heart disease may notice a further diminution in cardiac output. Special pacemakers (physiological pacemakers, see below) are being developed to overcome this problem.

What should pacemaker patients avoid doing?

They hardly need to avoid anything once the initial wound is well healed. Modern pacemakers are tough instruments in metal cases. They will not be damaged by minor trauma or affected by strenuous physical exertion. In the United Kingdom an ordinary driving licence can be regained 3 months after a pacemaker insertion has abolished the symptoms of a bradycardia. This can be an additional reason for pacing as even minor episodes of dizziness may lead to permanent loss of licence if they are not treated. Heavy goods vehicle or public service vehicles licences cannot be regained. Pacemaker patients can wear seat belts normally, though occasionally the belt may need adjusting if it is resting uncomfortably on the box.

Many anecdotal accounts are told of various forms of electrical or magnetic activity interfering with pacemaker function, especially the false inhibition of demand pacemakers. The problem is complicated by a lack of information from the manufacturers. This is partly because the exact design of a unit is a commercial secret, and partly because the largest market is the United States where the potential threat of legal action is always present if anything untoward should happen.

Modern pacemakers are very resistant to outside interference. It is best to avoid the metal detecting devices for screening passengers at airports; the pacemaker box will often set them off anyway. Similar devices are positioned at the exits of some libraries to stop book thefts. With programmable pacemakers the worry has been whether microwave ovens or other equipment could reset the pacing parameters. This is extremely unlikely and should not influence the patient's normal activities but, as a precaution, very close proximity to a microwave oven is best avoided.

The main difficulty sometimes lies in convincing the pacemaker patient and his relatives that restrictions are unnecessary. A feeling of 'taking things quietly' tends to persist though the principle reason for the operation was to get activities back to normal. Modern pacemakers are stronger than the bodies they are implanted in.

What are the pacemakers of the future?

Commercial competition between the large number of manufacturers means that the devices are continually being improved. With modern microelectronics almost anything can be done; the difficulty lies in knowing whether it benefits the patient.

For this reason the importance of 'physiological' pacing is still undecided. The standard pacemaker is available 'on demand' to pace the ventricles at a fixed rate. Physiological pacemakers can do a great deal more. They are complicated with separate 'wires' to the atria and ventricles. The 'wire' to the atria can pace these structures just before ventricular pacing to restore coordinated activity. Or the spontaneous atrial activity can be sensed and the ventricles paced immediately afterwards, allowing the heart rate to increase naturally with exercise. Some patients do benefit from these manoeuvres but whether all should be considered for physiological pacing in the future is uncertain. They do have snags such as more things to go wrong, increased cost, and reduced battery life.

Improvements in batteries should continue. Ideally a battery should last for the rest of a patient's life, but this is only true for elderly patients at present. A few nuclear-powered units were implanted in the 1970s but the necessary radiation screening makes them big and heavy. Today's lithium batteries last almost as long and nuclear units are no longer used.

A long term aim will be to make pacemakers unnecessary. They control the rate but they do not reverse the underlying heart disease. If we could find ways to prevent or repair the the damage to the conducting system, pacemakers could be relegated to the museums. However, there are no signs of this and for the forseeable future the number of patients with pacemakers will continue to rise.

7

Heart surgery

Heart surgery has glamour. Few could fail to be impressed by the bed-bound patient who is restored to normal life by the skill of a surgical team. But this image of success is not the complete picture. Operations are very effective in relieving some heart conditions and in helping others, but they cannot deal with many forms of heart disease. The public's expectations can be artificially high. The surgery is also dangerous. The risk has declined markedly in recent years but it is still there. In addition some discomfort and inconvenience is inevitable. Although a heart operation has changed from a rare event to one of the commonest forms of surgery in the last two decades, the problems cannot be ignored. This chapter is not intended to put people off having an operation. The benefits can be enormous and obvious. Afterwards many patients say that they wish they had been operated on earlier. But intelligent people know that there are potential snags as well.

The catalyst for the development of heart surgery was the introduction of cardiopulmonary bypass in the 1950s. Before then techniques had been limited by the inability to interrupt blood flow through the heart for more than a minute or two. With cardiopulmonary bypass, machines take over the functions of the heart and lungs, enabling the heart to be stopped and opened for much longer periods. All parts of the heart are now accessible to the surgeon, with sufficient time for repair or replacement as necessary.

Even today some procedures do not need cardiopulmonary bypass (often shortened to just 'bypass'). Operations on nearby vessels are readily performed with the heart beating normally. A patent ductus arteriosus (p.112) is ligated and a coarctation (p.115) repaired without interrupting the output from the heart. Sometimes a stenosed mitral valve (p.98) can be dilated without cardiopulmonary bypass. To do this, a special dilator is inserted through the left ventricle into the mitral valve and opened up to split the fibrosis without stopping the beating heart. The technique, known as closed mitral valvotomy, is not utilized very often today. The main disadvantage is the inadvertent creation of mitral incompetence. Surgeons often prefer to do an 'open' valvotomy under cardiopulmonary bypass where they can inspect the valve as they relieve the stenosis.

Most heart operations are done with cardiopulmonary bypass. The rest of this chapter will be concerned largely with these 'open-heart' procedures.

What is cardiopulmonary bypass?

The heart and lungs are isolated from the rest of the circulation which continues to function with the help of machines. The principles are quite simple (Figure 7.1). All the venous blood is drained off from the right atrium. The blood is passed through an artificial oxygenator which mimics the lungs by removing carbon dioxide and adding oxygen to the blood. It is then pumped back into the aorta at arterial pressure and flows through the body's circulation again. The heart itself is perfused with a special solution to arrest the chemistry of the heart muscle. This solution, known as cardioplegic solution, has two functions. One is to stop the heart and make the surgeon's task easier; the other is to preserve the heart muscle in a dormant state until the normal blood flows down the coronary arteries at the end of the operation. These aims may be assisted by cooling the heart at the same time.

Of course, the practical details of cardiopulmonary bypass are a good deal more complicated. A special group of technicians (perfusionists) are needed to use and maintain the machinery. The normal circulation is being continually modified by the nervous system. But this effect is lost with bypass, so constant measurements and mechanical adjustments are needed. Normal blood would clot in the machines, so it has to be anti-coagulated (p.70) with heparin. The temperature also has to be closely controlled.

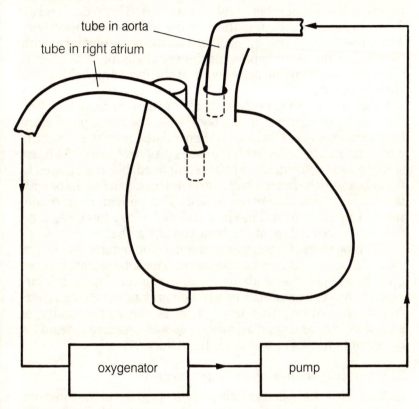

tube in aorta

tube in right atrium

oxygenator

pump

Figure 7.1. Cardiopulmonary bypass

Cardiopulmonary bypass can support the circulation satis-factorily for a time, but its duration is not unlimited. Surgeons like to limit total bypass time to about an hour and a half if possible, though partial support to the circulation may continue afterwards. A few procedures take longer and for these post-operative recovery is inevitably slower.

What happens during open-heart surgery?

The patient is usually sedated before being taken from the ward to the anaesthetic room close to the operating theatre. Anxiety makes the heart work harder. Sleep will be induced with an injection. Then a number of tubes are inserted into veins and an artery to monitor the circulation during and after the operation. The anaesthetized patient is placed on the operating table with the cardiopulmonary bypass machinery alongside. The chest is opened by splitting the breastbone at the front and holding the springy ribs apart.

Tubes are inserted into the right atrium and the aorta to collect the blood and return it to the body from the cardiopulmonary bypass machinery. The heart is then isolated from the rest of the circulation and stopped with the cardioplegic solution. The heart surgery is carried out. Once this is completed, blood is allowed to flow back into the heart which starts beating again, perhaps with the help of a small electric shock. The patient is gradually weaned off the bypass. The chest is closed, with wires being used to hold the two halves of the breastbone together.

The procedures for going on and coming off bypass take longer than the actual surgery on the heart. The total duration of an open-heart operation is about 4 hours or longer. The body's circulation has to be maintained satisfactorily under changing circumstances during this time. This is the responsibility of anaesthetists and perfusionists; a well-organized team is essential to the success of open-heart surgery.

What happens after open-heart surgery?

At the end of the operation the patient is moved to the intensive care area. A minimum time of several hours is needed to wake up from the long anaesthetic and during this period breathing will be supported by a machine (ventilator) blowing through a tube into the lungs. The patient gradually wakes up, though he will be unable to speak until the breathing tube has been removed. Detailed monitoring of the circulation continues in the immediate postoperative period. Patients and their relatives may be surprised at the number of tubes and leads necessary for this. Even after the simplest open-heart procedure three or more thin plastic tubes will be used to measure pressure in the circulation or to replace fluids. The heart rhythm will be monitored by electrode pads stuck to the front of the chest in a similar manner to a coronary care unit. A tube in the bladder will be used to measure urine flow. Two or three larger tubes come out of the chest for the first day or two. These are utilized to fully expand the lungs by removing any leaking air and to allow unwanted fluid to drain from the chest.

The speed of recovery from heart operations is very variable. Some patients may be in the intensive care area for less than 24 hours, while others need detailed monitoring or assisted breathing for several days. The hospital may have an 'intermediate care' area where monitoring can be continued on a less extensive basis. Back on the ordinary ward the patient is mobilized and drug treatment is adjusted. The stitches will be removed at about 10-14 days after the operation.

The length of stay in hospital depends not only on the speed of recovery but also the facilities available at home. A few patients might leave hospital as early as 10 days after the operation but most stay for 2-4 weeks. The return to full fitness takes longer. Most patients need 2 or 3 months before they get the maximum benefit of their operation. Then they often realize the full extent of their ill health before surgery. Heart symptoms often develop very gradually and their severity may not be appreciated until normality is restored.

What are the different types of open-heart surgery?

The large majority of these operations fall into three categories: valve surgery, coronary artery vein grafting, and operations for congenital heart disease.

Valve surgery

The simplest form of valve surgery is a dilatation of a stenosed mitral valve. As described earlier in this chapter, it can be done with cardiopulmonary bypass ('open') or without ('closed'). But most valve surgery involves removing the stenosed or incompetent valve and replacing it with an artificial one. If necessary the aortic, mitral, and tricuspid valves can all be replaced in a single operation.

In the past a wide variety of synthetic valves or preserved human and animal valves have been utilized. Nowadays only two types are used with any degree of frequency. These are pig valves suspended on a frame (for example, Hancock and Carpentier-Edwards valves) or entirely synthetic models made from metal and plastic (for example, Bjork-Shiley and Starr-Edwards valves). The modified pig valves have the advantage over synthetic valves of being less liable to provoke blood clotting, but the synthetic valves are sometimes more resilient.

Artificial valves are much better than the diseased valves they replace, but they are not quite as good as a normal valve. It is always hoped that an artificial valve will last for the remainder of the patient's life. Valves have been replaced in significant numbers for the last 20 years and many of the early models are still working satisfactorily. But some have had to be replaced. The artificial valves used today are tougher and most will never need to be changed. But, as with any mechanical structure, some will go wrong eventually. The patients are seen from time to time in the outpatient clinic so that the early signs of any malfunction can be picked up.

With synthetic valves precautions are taken to prevent clot formation. The blood has a natural tendency to clot when it comes into contact with a synthetic surface. Clots could obstruct the working of the valve or embolize to distant parts of the body (p.103). This tendency is controlled by a long-term anti-coagulation with a drug called warfarin. This technique has already been described for patients with mitral stenosis (p.104). Most synthetic valve replacements need indefinite warfarin therapy. With the modified pig valves the warfarin can be stopped a month or two after the operation when healing is complete.

Coronary artery vein grafting

This has become one of the commonest of all surgical operations in Europe and North America. A superficial vein is removed from the leg and used to take blood past obstructions in the coronary arteries. One end of the vein is joined to the aorta and the other to the artery beyond the blockage (Figure 7.2). A pre-operative coronary arteriogram (p.39) is essential to demonstrate the exact position of the obstructions. The indications for the operation have been mentioned in Chapter 4. The loss of the leg vein is of no practical importance as most of the blood from the leg does not travel in the superficial veins. Several alternative routes provide a satisfactory venous return. A minor degree of ankle swelling may be present for a time. Anticoagulation with warfarin may be required for the first few weeks postoperatively.

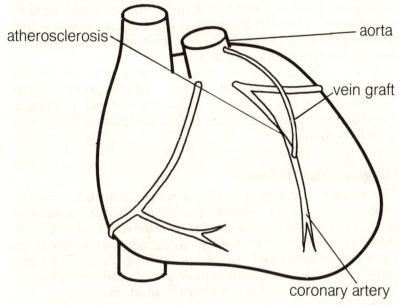

Figure 7.2. Coronary artery bypass

Vein grafting is certainly an effective method of bypassing obstructions, but it does have limitations. Only disease in the larger arteries can be treated. If multiple narrowings are found it may be impossible to bypass them all. Restoration of blood supply will not affect infarcted areas of the heart where the muscle is already destroyed and replaced by a scar. The operation will not stop any progression of the coronary artery disease, which may eventually undo the benefits by creating fresh obstructions. The vein grafts themselves can become diseased. Vein grafting is not a panacea for all forms of coronary artery disease.

Having said this, vein grafting is an excellent treatment for intractable angina in selected patients. About three patients out of four will have their angina abolished and most of the others will be improved. As discussed in Chapter 4, it may also reduce the chances of future myocardial infarctions in some subjects, but in many it does not alter the long-term risk to any significant extent. Psychologically, the attractions of 'doing something positive' can be enormous, but the snags need to appreciated. This can be difficult in countries where a free market philosophy in medicine is combined with much higher fees for surgery than for drug treatment.

A few patients who are rendered symptom free by the operation find that the angina returns when the grafts block or the coronary artery disease worsens. Further vein grafting is possible in some but it becomes technically more difficult with each operation.

Congenital heart disease

The surgery of congenital defects ranges from fairly simple procedures such as closure of a patent ductus arteriosus (p. 112) to complex operations to reverse the effects of an absent chamber or major vessel. Some abnormalities can be corrected, some can be alleviated, and a few are inoperable. The eight commonest congenital defects have been described in Chapter 5; they are all amenable to surgery in most children.

Cardiopulmonary bypass in children is based on the same principles as in adults. The technical problems of dealing with such small patients can be formidable but babies may be operated on within a few hours of birth if necessary. However, surgery at this age is kept to a minimum with complete correction of the defect often being left till later. Fortunately children are very resilient and usually recover from an operation much faster than adults.

What is a 'cabbage' operation?

This is doctors' slang for coronary artery vein grafting. The operation is sometimes called coronary artery bypass grafting and the initials of this term (CABG) are pronounced as 'cabbage'.

What are the side-effects of open-heart surgery?

Surgery is not an easy option. A certain amount of discomfort and inconvenience is inevitable with all procedures. In addition heart operations are often preceded by cardiac catheterization (p.37) which in itself is a small operation, even though it is performed with a local anaesthetic.

After an open-heart operation, chest pain is one of the most prominent sensations. In addition to any discomfort from the wound down the front of the chest, pushing the ribs apart to gain access may result in some residual pain. In most patients the chest wound heals quickly and the pain is much better within a few days. Surprisingly, a leg wound from a vein removal for grafting may be more troublesome than the chest wound. An occasional chest wound becomes infected and healing is delayed. A few patients have a mild degree of discomfort in the ribs and surrounding muscles for weeks or months after surgery. This resolves spontaneously in due course.

The work of breathing is done by a machine during and immediately after the operation. The patient is unable to cough and clear unwanted secretions during this period. The result may be a chest infection, particularly in smokers. The infection can be readily treated but it may delay recovery. Blood transfusions are an essential part of the operative procedure so a blood transmitted infection is a possibility; but this is very rare with modern transfusion services.

During cardiopulmonary bypass care is taken to ensure that solid matter or air does not get into the blood. Either could temporarily block an artery somewhere in the body. Blood clot is the commonest form of solid matter, so the patient is anticoagulated throughout the procedure. In addition the blood is filtered as it passes through the bypass pump. Occasionally very small particles squeeze through the filters and pass to the brain, producing transient visual and other disturbances in the postoperative period. These effects pass off in time.

What are the risks of open-heart surgery?

All operations have some degree of risk. Even a trivial procedure like removing an ingrowing toe nail will very occasionally go wrong. Open-heart surgery is complex and inevitably carries a small, but significant, risk. In the past the chance of not coming through the operation was quite high, perhaps one in five in the early days. Nowadays the degree of risk is much less and is similar to other forms of major surgery. It also has to be balanced against the risk of *not* having an operation which may be greater.

It is impossible to put a precise figure on the degree of risk. It depends partly on the type of operation. The dangers of closing a moderate sized atrial septal defect (p. 111) in a fit adolescent are very small, probably no more than removing the same patient's inflamed appendix. Emergency surgery in a sick new-born baby carries a high risk, though it may be life saving.

The severity of the heart disease is also important. Coronary artery vein grafting can be done on some patients with a mortality risk of less than one per cent (that is 99 per cent of the patients come through the operation); other patients with severe heart damage due to the coronary artery disease might have a ten times greater risk for the same operation. The general state of the patient's health is another factor. An aortic valve replacement in a young patient might have a risk of 2 per cent (98 per cent come through), but it will be considerably larger for a man of 70 years with bad lungs and narrowed arteries to the brain.

The risks of not having the operation must also be considered. In many patients the hazards of an uncorrected defect are greater than the dangers of an operation. This is apart from the abolition of symptoms that the operation may bring. Fortunately, it is uncommon to have to balance the risks of surgery against just the chances of symptomatic improvement. The defects which cause the most symptoms are often the problems which need surgery to improve the outlook. When the dangers of surgery are less than the dangers of not having surgery, the true risk of an operation is nothing.

Does surgery remove the risk of endocarditis?

On the whole, it does not; sometimes it increases it. As discussed in Chapter 5 many congenital defects or diseased valves can get infected (endocarditis). A common source is bacteria from the mouth gaining access to the blood stream as a result of poor dental hygiene or teeth extraction. In these patients surgery does not remove the need for precautions against endocarditis such as regular dental checks and antibiotic therapy immed- iately before teeth extractions or other procedures that might induce gum bleeding. On the contrary, it normally makes them even more important. An infection on an artificial valve is difficult to eradicate, as the valve does not have a blood supply of its own and so a high concentration of antibiotic at the site of infection may not be obtainable.

The exceptions to this are a few congenital defects which can be completely corrected by surgery. Closure of a patent ductus arteriosus (p.112) abolishes the risk of endocarditis. Indeed, the operation was first introduced to treat such an infection in the preantibiotic era. Repair of a simple ventricular defect (p.112) reduces the chances of getting endocarditis later.

What is a coronary angioplasty?

Coronary angioplasty is a new technique for surgically dilating a narrowed coronary artery. It is done in the X-ray department on a conscious patient. With the help of X-ray screening, a deflated balloon is passed up to the heart from the groin artery and positioned at the narrowing in the coronary artery. The balloon is inflated suddenly, disrupting the atherosclerotic obstruction and increasing the size of the lumen. The artery is still diseased, but the procedure can usually restore normal blood flow down it.

With a single major coronary artery obstruction, angioplasty is an attractive alternative to vein grafting. A chest incision is not required. The technique is done under local anaesthetic, so recovery is fast, and the patient can often go home within a few days. If necessary, angioplasty can be repeated more readily than open-heart surgery.

Unfortunately, most patients have multiple coronary artery narrowings which cannot be dealt with by angioplasty at the present time. In addition the risks of angioplasty are very similar to the risks of vein grafting, so it is not a safer alternative in spite of its apparent simplicity. Occasionally, the procedure worsens the coronary artery disease and the patient has to be taken immediately to the operating theatre for a vein graft. Angioplasty will be performed with increasing frequency in the years ahead, but it is unlikely to be an alternative to vein grafting in the majority of patients.

Why are there waiting lists for heart surgery?

A short wait can be advantageous to the patient if his condition is stable. Arrangements for the operation can be made calmly and thoroughly. Any non-cardiac medical problems can be properly assessed. The blood for transfusion will be carefully cross-matched and a plentiful supply obtained.

But in the United Kingdon the wait may be months or even years. In a sense this is a tribute to heart surgery. More defects can be dealt with and many patients are considered for surgery in spite of advancing age or other problems. The number of operations performed has risen sharply in the last ten years, but the increase has not been sufficient to keep down waiting lists. The structure of the National Health Service is such that anticipation of future needs is almost impossible; the Service can only react when the extra demand is already present. Yet it is only through the same National Health Service that thousands of people with modest incomes have been able to have heart surgery. The operations are not cheap; each costs several thousands of pounds. But in terms of saving lives and symptom relief, heart surgery is one of the most effective forms of surgery.

Apart from the patient's discomfort while waiting with uncorrected symptoms, the main worry is the potential risk attached to remaining on a list for several months. Some problems such as simple congenital defects have no immediate dangers and waiting is no more than a nuisance. Other abnormalities clearly have a major risk while unoperated and they will be done as urgent cases within a few days or weeks. The difficulty is the large number of patients within these extremes who are not particularly at risk, but nevertheless could deteriorate if the wait is long. Within this group it is hard to pick out those that might suffer from the delay. Nobody should wait longer than 2 or 3 months without good reason, but in Britain we are a long way from this modest aim.

In the long term the general public's perception of need will determine the resources made available for heart surgery.

Unfortunately, people are becoming used to waiting for these operations. A delay of several months for cancer surgery would raise an immediate outcry, but a similar wait for a heart operation is accepted. Lists are still growing and painful decisions about priorities for surgery will have to be made unless help can be provided.

Is there an upper age limit for heart surgery?

The general state of health is more important than a precise age. 'Biological age' is a better guide than the calendar. Some units with rapidly increasing waiting lists use an age range as a guide to priorities, but in general there is no strict limit above which surgery is impossible. In practice many patients over 70, and some under, have other medical problems which make surgery riskier and less successful. An occasional patient in the late 70s has had a good result from surgery but this is rare.

How is heart transplantation performed?

The first requirement is the donation of a suitable heart. Young people who have been killed in road accidents or other traumatic events are the best donors. In Britain the heart is removed at the hospital where the donor dies and is brought to the hospital where the transplant is to take place. During transport the heart is preserved in a dormant state by an infusion of a special solution known as cardioplegic solution. Similar solutions are used to preserve hearts during ordinary open-heart surgery.

As the new heart is being collected, the patient's chest is being opened and cardiopulmonary bypass is instituted. The old heart is removed and the new one inserted. The new healthy heart usually restarts beating easily and the patient is soon in the intensive care area.

In terms of its immediate effects on the patient a transplant is similar to other open-heart procedures. The patient usually wakes up within hours and a prompt recovery ensues. Within a few days the patient often feels better than he has done for years. The surgery is not particularly difficult, though a considerable amount of organization is needed to ensure that the new heart is collected simultaneously with the preparation of the patient several miles away.

The hardest part for the patient and his doctors is the constant assessment and antirejection treatment which continues for the rest of the patient's life. Without treatment the body's natural defences would recognize the new heart as 'foreign' and reject it. The rejection can be controlled by drugs, but the inhibition of the defence mechanisms makes the patient vulnerable to severe infections. The treatment is a continuous balancing act between abolishing rejection, but not damping down the defences so much that bacteria and other organisms can produce dangerous infections. The drugs are kept to the minimum doses needed to control rejection, so it is important that impending rejection can be diagnosed early to allow for a brief increase in the dosage before the heart is permanently damaged. Some of the findings in examination are a help in diagnosis and the size of deflections on the electrocardiogram may be an indication of early rejection.

To confirm suspected rejection an instrument (bioptome) is passed into the heart through a vein and a small scraping (biopsy) is removed from inside of the right ventricle for microscopic examination. This simple procedure is repeated frequently in the early postoperative period.

Who might need a transplant?

The operation is confined to men and women under 55 years with chronic heart failure which cannot be controlled by other means. The failure is usually due to coronary artery disease or a cardiomyopathy (p.125). But many in this group are not considered for the operation. The patient must have no other significant medical problem. He must be ill enough for the risk to be worth taking, but not so ill that he cannot wait until a donor heart is available. In particular he (or she) must be psychologically resilient. The indefinite postoperative treatment is hard. The first month or more is spent in isolation to reduce the risk of infection. Several drugs must be taken every day for years, and repeated examinations and tests are required. The patient must be able to tolerate this for the rest of his life.

Is transplantation worth while?

The early efforts at heart transplantation in the late 1960s were almost a complete failure. Today's results are better, but it is still a very high-risk procedure. About 70 per cent of patients survive the first year and about 60 per cent are alive at three years. This may sound disappointing but it has to be compared with the outlook for similar patients who do not have a transplant. Without surgery only 10-20 per cent survive for a year.

In Britain attention has focused on the cost of each operation. It is not cheap, with costs of about £20,000 in addition to the cost of a routine open-heart operation. Opponents of transplantation argue that the money could be better spent on more conventional forms of treatment or prevention. Enthusiasts remark that other medical procedures are more expensive or less successful (or both) and transplantation has only been singled out for attack because it is in the public eye. They also claim that without transplantation the costs of looking after a patient in severe chronic heart failure are not negligible. The topic will be debated for some time to come. But the number of potential recipients of a heart transplantation is relatively small — only a few hundred a year for the whole of Britain. Taken on a national basis the financial implications are minimal.

8

Prevention of heart disease

Prevention of heart disease is a popular subject. Methods of controlling the commonest form of death in the western world should claim everybody's attention. But it is not an easy topic. The seeds of coronary artery disease are probably sown a decade or more before any illness appears: this makes scientific investigation difficult. Also the field tends to attract enthusiasts for one particular aspect. In many ways their zeal is commendable but they can blunt the message to the general public by saying different things. Even some experts fail to distinguish clearly between what they know is happening and what they hope is happening. Articles, books, press reports, and television shows pour forth to the confusion of the non-expert. One day low-fat foods are important, the next day more fibre in the diet is the thing, and the day after less sugar is essential. In this chapter we will try to pick a way through, hopefully remembering the difference between facts and assumptions at all times.

In a brief article in a popular newspaper or magazine getting rid of heart disease can seem simple. But we only have to look around us to see that the problem has not been solved; it has yet to show much sign of fading away. Oversimplification can make anything straightforward. For example, 'heart disease' is regarded as synonymous with coronary artery disease. Atherosclerosis in the coronary arteries may be the commonest form of heart disease but valve defects, rhythm disturbances, and congenital abnormalities cannot be ignored.

Many of these non-atherosclerotic problems are not preventable with our present state of knowledge. But some are and have already been mentioned in the relevant chapters. The incidence of valve infections (endocarditis) can be reduced by appropriate dental care (p.108). Embolization of blood clots from around stenosed mitral valves can be controlled by warfarin therapy (p.103). Some congenital heart defects can be avoided by immunizing potential mothers against German measles (p.110). These aspects of prevention will not be discussed further in this chapter which will deal exclusively with coronary artery disease in its different forms.

What is meant by prevention?

Nobody claims that we can prevent coronary artery disease in the sense of getting rid of it completely. Prevention in this context means reducing the incidence. If every known risk factor was corrected for each person in Britain, people would still get coronary artery disease. But even in this modified sense prevention has two different meanings. It can be applied to stopping heart disease in previously *healthy people* — primary prevention. It also means reducing the risk of progression of heart disease in *patients* who have already had angina or a myocardial infarction — secondary prevention. We often hope that measures shown to be effective for primary prevention will help in secondary prevention (or vice versa), but there is no automatic reason why this should not be true.

We also have to consider what exactly we are preventing. We have already seen in Chapter 4 that the three major manifestations of coronary artery disease (angina, myocardial infarction, and sudden death) overlap, but are not due to the same mechanisms. Angina is normally produced by insufficient blood flow through a narrow coronary artery. Myocardial infarction is largely due to a thrombotic obstruction of a major artery. Sudden death is often produced by electrical instability secondary to a diseased ventricle. Although coronary artery disease is a major factor in all, they each have a different precipitating event. A preventative measure might reduce the risk of all three manifestations, or it might affect only one.

Can coronary artery disease be prevented?

Certainly some of it can be prevented, though we do not know how much. One of the most compelling pieces of evidence for this is the wide variation in incidence among different populations. These populations can be represented by countries: Figure 8.1 shows that the death rate in men from coronary artery disease is three times higher in Scotland than in Italy and ten times higher in Japan. Different social groups in the same country also illustrate the varying occurrence of the disease. Amongst men under 45 years in Britain, the death rate from this disease is twice as high in unskilled manual workers (social class V) than in professional and managerial men (class I). Preventable causes must be responsible for at least some of these differences. In developing countries the bulk of the people are very poor and rarely get angina or a myocardial infarction, while these diseases are common in the few who earn money and develop westernized tastes.

Additional evidence for the ability to prevent heart disease is a changing incidence within one country. The most quoted example comes from the United States which had a 20 per cent fall in deaths from coronary artery disease from 1968 to 1976 after a steady rise in the years before. Overall, Britain has failed to show a similar decline, but in the 1960s British doctors had a decrease in deaths from this cause, probably as a result of reduced cigarette smoking. It seems clear that the number of people developing heart disease can be reduced, but experts may differ about the precise methods for achieving this.

Why are we uncertain about some methods of preventing heart disease

Superficially, it is amazing that doctors and scientists can invest so much time and money in finding out about prevention and still be uncertain about some of the basic points. But the work is difficult for a number of reasons. The seeds of coronary artery disease are sown decades before the heart disease is found. Few investigations have the resources to continue for more than ten years, which is only a fraction of a lifetime. Also people are not laboratory animals. They cannot be fed on the same food each day, nor do their habits remain constant for long periods of time.

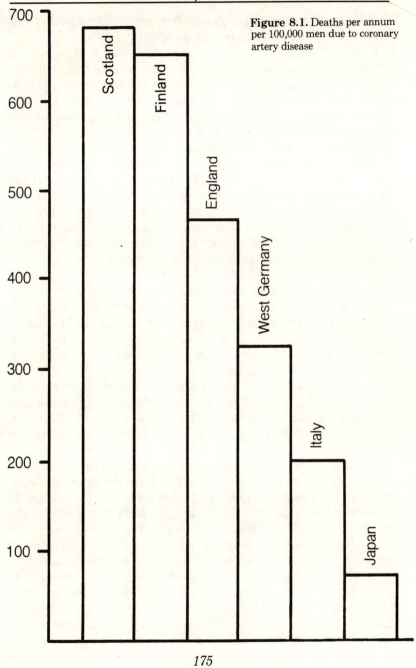

Figure 8.1. Deaths per annum per 100,000 men due to coronary artery disease

To get significant results large numbers are needed and then it is hard to keep track of the people involved.

Even when the results of a study are reported their interpretation may be controversial. The fundamental problem, which will be referred to several times in this chapter, is that association is not the same as cause. The incidence of heart disease in many countries can show a close *association* to the sale of television sets; they both show an increase in the last 20 years. But nobody has yet suggested that watching television directly *causes* heart trouble. The mere observation that, for example, men who do little exercise are more likely to have a myocardial infarction than those who indulge in physical training does not by itself prove that lack of exercise is one of the causes of infarction. It could be, but there are alternative explanations. One might be that the physically active men smoke less and this is the real reason for their reduced risk of heart disease.

To establish that lack of exercise was a cause of the increased rate of heart disease in these men further studies are required. One method would be to place a number of men at a factory into two identical groups and then persuade one group to exercise regularly and the other to continue as before. The two groups would otherwise be identical in terms of smoking habits and other risk factors. After several years the incidence of myocardial infarction in the two groups would be reviewed; a significant reduction in the exercise group would help to establish that lack of exercise is one factor in the cause of infarction. Unfortunately this type of study is very difficult to organize and complete.

Another problem is the interpretation of negative results. If this group of exercising men is found to have the same incidence of infarction as the non-exercising men, three interpretations are possible. One is that the study design was faulty. Perhaps the exercise was not sufficiently vigorous, or the non-exercising group learnt about the possible benefits of exercise and started physical training on their own initiative. A second possibility is that the number of men studied was not big enough to demonstrate a small but definite benefit. Neither of these conclusions disprove the suggestion that exercise is good for the heart; they just leave the question open. A third interpretation is that lack of exercise is indeed not a factor in the genesis of an infarction. This type of study is very hard to repeat, so arguments about the correct interpretation can continue for years after the figures are presented.

Once concrete results have been obtained, it must be remembered that the conclusions only apply to the problem being studied. Interventions which reduce the risk of healthy people getting heart disease (primary prevention) may not be effective once the patient has angina (secondary prevention). Something that helped with angina may not influence the chances of having an infarction. Techniques of reducing heart disease on Scotland (high incidence) may be irrelelvant to Japan (low incidence). However, a certain amount of well-informed judgement has to be applied. If everything had to be demonstrated for every social class in every country with every manifestation of coronary artery disease, the number of studies would have to be enormous before any action could be taken. From time to time, results have to be extrapolated on the basis of 'it seems reasonable' until further information is made available.

This approach to the assessment of prevention may seem over-critical. But the general public is flooded with advice on the subject, some of it contradictory, and it is important to appreciate the firmness of each piece of evidence. Modification of personal habits over a period of many years is not easy and needs to be based on solid foundations.

Are all risk factors important in the avoidance of heart disease?

The concept of risk factors was introduced in Chapter 4. Several factors are associated with an increased incidence of coronary artery disease. But some cannot be modified and so are irrelevant to this chapter. Being male and getting older are both strongly associated, but neither can be readily changed. A strong family history of coronary artery disease is another risk factor which cannot be altered. The other factors can be modified to some degree, so they are *potential* targets in the search for means of reducing the risk of coronary artery disease.

Smoking

Avoidance of smoking will always be an important manoeuvre in the prevention of heart disease. Smoking is a strong risk factor and it is also one that can, in theory, be corrected overnight.

Is cigarette smoking associated with coronary artery disease?

Yes, cigarette smoking is strongly associated. Smoking 20 cigarettes a day trebles the chance of dying from a myocardial infarction before the age of 50. Or put in another way, each minute spent smoking, on average, is associated with a minute's less life expectancy. There is no safe level of consumption. Even a few cigarettes each day is harmful and the greater the number the greater the risk.

Does stopping smoking reduce the risk of heart disease?

The association between smoking and heart disease is so strong that it is difficult to argue against smoking being a factor in the creation of coronary artery disease. But additional evidence can be provided by observations that stopping smoking reduces the risk when compared to similar individuals who carry on. After stopping, the extra risk is halved in about 2 years and disappears completely after 10 years. So it is never too late to stop. As mentioned already, doctors in Britain have sharply reduced their smoking in the last 25 years and are the only occupational group in the country to show a marked fall in the incidence of coronary artery disease.

Does stopping smoking reduce the risk of recurrence of an infarction?

Yes, patients who stop smoking after an infarction have less than half the chance of developing another infarction or other complications than those who continue.

Why are cigarettes harmful?

Several mechanisms seem to be involved, though they are not completely understood. The nicotine in the smoke encourages the release of catecholamines which can overstimulate the heart and worsen the effects of any coronary artery disease. The nicotine may also enhance the formation of atherosclerosis, the underlying cause of the narrowed coronary artery.

Cigarette smoke also has a high carbon monoxide content. Carbon monoxide is a gas formed by incomplete combustion and can prove fatal when produced in large quantities by defective gas appliances in poorly ventilated rooms. The gas binds to the haemoglobin in the red cells of the blood, reducing their ability to carry oxygen. This will aggravate the effects of the narrowed coronary arteries. The carbon monoxide also increases the stickiness of small blood cells called platelets. Platelets have a major role in clot formation, so increased stickiness will promote clotting in the coronary arteries. Nicotine may also increase stickiness.

The relative importance of these and other mechanisms is uncertain. But it is clear that inhaling the smoke increases the dangers considerably. Smoking the cigarette right down to the butt also seems to magnify the risks. This is because some of the noxious substances from the far end of the cigarette are absorbed in the end closest to the mouth, but are then released again as more of the cigarette is smoked. One suggestion to explain the recent fall in deaths in the United States is that, with increasing affluence and cheap cigarettes there, smokers are throwing away the cigarette after smoking half or less.

What other diseases are promoted by smoking?

The dreary catalogue is already familiar to most smokers. Lung cancer is very strongly linked; indeed it is quite rare in non-smokers. Nevertheless the extra deaths from heart disease due to smoking are about four times as numerous as those secondary to lung cancer. Chronic lung damage in the form of bronchitis and emphysema is another well-known hazard. It can represent years of debilitation for tens of thousands of men in Britain. Attention has recently focused on the reduced birth weight and increased incidence of stillbirths amongst babies whose mothers smoke during pregnancy. Smokers also have an increased risk of cancer of the mouth and gullet.

Is pipe or cigar smoking harmful?

The number of pipe and cigar smokers is small compared to cigarette smokers. So the evidence for their harmful effect is less definite. But there is nothing to indicate that they are basically any safer. Fortunately, lifelong pipe smokers often do not inhale and may spend more time fiddling with their pipe than actually smoking it. So their extra risk of heart disease may not be great. But cigarette smokers who inhale will usually continue to do so when they switch to a pipe. If they do the hazards may not be altered much.

Some evidence hints that heavy cigar smoking may be more dangerous than heavy cigarette smoking. But economics rules out this risk for most people.

Is there a 'safe' cigarette?

Tobacco substitutes had a brief flare of publicity a few years ago. They were promoted as a safe form of smoking. But no attempt was made to prove this and they could have been as dangerous as tobacco. Fortunately, they were unpopular and soon disappeared from the shops.

Are low-tar cigarettes safer?

The tar content of cigarettes does seem to be responsible for some (but not all) of their ill-effects and a switch to a low-tar brand is helpful as long as the number smoked is not increased. But many smokers find that they have to smoke more low-tar cigarettes to get the same 'satisfaction'. An increase will cancel the benefits. The best solution is to stop smoking, not to change brands.

What is 'passive smoking'? *ind.*

Indoors, non-smokers have to breathe some of the smoke produced by other people's cigarettes. Attention has been drawn to the possible health hazards of this passive smoking. Young children and babies who passively inhale their parent's smoke have a higher incidence of chest infections than those in non-smoking families, The adult, non-smoking, close relatives of smokers may have an increased risk of heart disease, but the evidence is not quite so good. Non-smokers are probably more worried by the runny eyes, cough, and undesirable smell which they are often subjected to by smokers.

The unhealthy example set to children is another negative aspect of smoking. Children will tend to follow the habits of their parents and other influential adults, such as teachers. Once 'hooked', they may find stopping difficult.

Is smoking decreasing in Britain?

The answer to this question will vary depending on whether we are considering the number of people smoking, the number of cigarettes sold, or the amount of tobacco taxed by the Treasury. In general the number of people smoking has declined sharply in the last few years and non-smokers are now in a majority of nearly two to one over smokers; though this has yet to be appreciated by all those providing seating accommodation in restaurants, cinemas and many other public places. But smokers are tending to smoke more, so the number of cigarettes and the quantity of tobacco show a smaller reduction.

These general statements disguise marked differences in habits within the conventional five social classes. Smoking in class I (professional and managerial) has declined markedly so only one person in five in this group now smokes. The number of smokers in class V (unskilled manual workers) has only decreased slightly, largely due to some women in this group taking up the habit. The variations in deaths from ischaemic heart disease and lung disease between these two classes reflect these differences in smoking habits. The reasons for the variation are not completely understood — they could be very helpful in finding the best method to stop smoking. A repetitive, boring, occupation could encourage smoking. Educational differences might be important.

Should cigarette advertising be banned?

Cigarette smoking is the major preventable public health hazard in Britain. In the past, major public health problems have been quickly dealt with by measures such as improved sanitation or vaccination. Many doctors have criticized the lack of effective action to reduce smoking, in particular the few curbs on advertising. The money spent on antismoking campaigns is paltry compared to the amount used for advertising.

The tobacco industry has some powerful allies. It provides employment for many people. The tax on cigarettes raises a large amount of money — but much of it is used by the Health Service to deal with the effects of smoking. The companies make contributions to political parties and employ members of Parliament as advisors. So far advertising restrictions have depended on voluntary agreements with the companies — that is, agreements that do not influence sales to any great extent. The restrictions can be circumvented. For example, a ban on television advertising has been partly negated by sponsorship of sports events, which are then shown on television.

Sooner or later this problem will have to be faced squarely. In the long term jobs cannot be protected, government revenue retained and sports events sponsored by manufacturing and selling a product that kills thousands of people every year. At the very least compulsory restrictions of cigarette promotion will have to be implemented.

How do I stop smoking?

Smokers are rarely short of advice on this topic, some of it contradictory. Smokers represent a cross-section of society with all its wide variations. The techniques described here have helped many, but they will not be suitable for everybody. Three stages are needed — get the facts, plan the strategy, and carry it out.

Get the facts

The main reasons for giving up are already familiar to most smokers and have been outlined earlier in this chapter. For each smoker one reason may be pertinent, such as avoiding damaging the baby in the womb, not setting a bad example to the children, or because a doctor has strongly advised it on medical grounds. Do not forget that 20 cigarettes a day is costing a smoker £250 or more a year in the United Kingdon. Remember that the smell of cigarette smoke can make you unnattractive to non-smokers. A strong reason for giving up can be very helpful in the first difficult day or two after stopping.

Any lingering doubts or rationalizations for not stopping should be anticipated. It is never too late. The extra risk of heart disease falls sharply on quitting and is halved within two years. Putting on weight after stopping is a major worry to some people. The average weight gain is $1\frac{1}{2}$ — 2 kilos, though it may take the form of a greater initial increase followed by a fall. This degree of weight gain will hardly be noticed. The health risks of putting on even a lot of weight after stopping are far less than the risks of smoking. Remember that a major reason for putting on weight is that people feel better with an improved sense of taste; so they eat more. The increased appetite can be controlled.

Stopping is not easy. If it was, you would have done it already. With sufficient motivation everybody can give up smoking. If smokers are placed in a different environment with no possibility of smoking, such as in hospital coronary care unit, they rarely have any difficulty in stopping. Do not underestimate your own determination. You can win a contest between your health, appearance, and wellbeing, and a small piece of roast vegetable matter wrapped in paper.

Plan the strategy

The first decision is whether to stop suddenly or to reduce the number of cigarettes gradually. The advantages of stopping suddenly are that it is quicker and probably more effective. Most of the craving for cigarettes disappears within four or five days and has gone completely after two or three weeks. Reducing gradually may seem easier, but it can take months. Sustaining enthusiasm for this long period can be hard; halving the number of cigarettes is relatively simple, but then it becomes very difficult and few people manage to give up smoking by this method. Stopping suddenly has a higher chance of success.

The next step is to define the reasons for smoking so that methods can be devised to satisfy these needs during the first few crucial days after stopping. Some smokers derive most pleasure from handling the cigarettes and watching the smoke; fiddling with a pencil or doodling might be a substitute. Others find that smoking is a way of sitting still and thinking without any embarrassment; reading a book or watching television could fill this gap. Young women may need a cigarette to maintain social poise; they must avoid awkward moments in the first few days. Some smokers like the feel of something in their mouths; sucking an empty pipe or chewing gum can fulfil this need. All these groups of smokers should be able to give up without undue difficulty if they are really motivated, as their dependency on cigarettes is limited.

Other smokers are more reliant on cigarettes. Smoking is a habit rather than an addiction, but some people need a cigarette for stimulation while others, paradoxically, find it relaxing. The former must find alternative means of stimulation. More exercise or an increase in cups of tea and coffee may help. People who require a smoke to prevent tension can devise alternative relaxation techniques. Some find yoga or meditation helpful. A simple method is to sit down (or lie down if possible). Starting at the feet, each set of muscles is contracted and then relaxed in turn. The process spreads up to and includes the face muscles. Then let all the muscles relax for a time. This sort of techniquue may only be needed in the first days after stopping.

Carry it out

Once the broad strategy has been decided upon, set a date in advance for giving up. If you mostly smoke at work, make it the beginning of a holiday period. If you get most pleasure from a cigarette while relaxing, do it on a working Monday morning. Two or three people giving up together will strengthen each other's resolve. It may be helpful to tell your friends in advance but some find secrecy easier. On the evening before stopping a small ritual of burning the remaining cigarettes and throwing away a lighter can be useful. A stay in hospital for whatever reason is a relatively easy time to stop.

Doctors can give some practical assistance, but there is no substitute for personal motivation. Antismoking clinics are available in some areas. A few people find hypnotism helpful. Nicotine-containing tablets (Nicorette) may be sucked in the first few weeks. They are useful in those smokers who cannot tolerate the sudden loss of nicotine stimulation. At present in Britain they are only available on private prescription. This has caused some amusement in medical circles: tablets containing nicotine are thought to be too dangerous to be bought over the counter while cigarettes with more nicotine plus additional toxic substances can be purchased by any adult. The nicotine tablets are tailed off over a few weeks. But none of these aids are effective unless the smoker is determined to give up. Motivation is the key to stopping smoking.

Two or 3 weeks after stopping successful quitters find that it was easier than expected and wonder why they did not do it before. Some ex-smokers find that they are never tempted to smoke again, but others have to maintain some vigilance. The important point is never to smoke a cigarette again. After even one the craving can be unbearable. Putting aside the money that would have been spent on cigarettes and using it for something special may help. Telling everybody that you have stopped should prevent them offering you one.

If you are unsuccessful do not despair. It is always worth having another effort later. Many ex-smokers have needed several attempts before finally stopping. In the meantime keep the number of cigarettes down to a minimum and switch to a low-tar brand. Try again in a few months' time.

High blood pressure

High blood pressure (hypertension) has already been discussed in Chapter 4. This section will concentrate on the potential benefits of blood pressure control in the prevention of heart trouble. The methods of treatment have aready been described on page 90 and will not be repeated.

Does hypertension cause coronary artery disease?

It is certainly associated with coronary artery disease. As mentioned on page 79 blood pressure is recorded as two values, the maximum (systolic) and the minimum (diastolic) pressures. The pressures are expressed as being equivalent to the pressure generated by a column of so many millimetres of mercury and written together (135/80, for example). Elevations in both the systolic and diastolic values are associated with an increased risk of coronary artery disease. The higher the pressure, the greater is the risk.

But association is not the same as cause. An important piece of evidence for hypertension's direct influence on coronary artery disease would be to show abolition of the risk by control of the raised pressure. Treatment certainly reduces the risk of strokes kidney damage, and hypertensive heart failure. It can improve symptoms produced by pre-existing heart disease such as angina. But several studies on hypertensive people who are fit and well at the start of treatment have failed to show a reduction in the incidence of subsequent coronary artery disease. These surveys were often performed with drugs which are rarely used now, so they may not reveal the complete picture. Today's better treatment could improve long-term blood pressure control.

Some evidence is coming through that the incidence of coronary artery disease can be reduced by treating hypertension, but it is not yet definite. So, although hypertension is associated with this form of heart disease, we cannot say for certain that the raised pressure is a cause.

Why do we use antihypertensive treatment in asymptomatic subjects, if it does not prevent coronary artery disease?

The major reason is that treatment of moderate to severe hypertension (that is diastolic pressures above about 100mm) has been clearly shown to save lives. The therapy produces a marked reduction in the risk of having a stroke and also diminishes the chances of kidney damage. It will also reduce the complications of coronary artery disease and other forms of heart disease. We do not yet know whether the treatment of mild hypertension (diastolic pressure 90—100 millimetres) saves lives. It may do and large-scale drug trials are currently under way to resolve this problem.

The control of hypertension *may* decrease the risk of developing heart disease, though we have not yet demonstrated it unequivocably. Earlier studies may have used the wrong drugs or may have not included enough people. The problems of interpreting a negative result in the field of prevention have already been discussed earlier in the chapter.

How does somebody know that his blood pressure is raised?

Usually, he does not know. Raised pressure rarely produces any symptoms until complications have occurred. For this reason everybody should have their blood pressure checked at least every three years. The measurement (p.87) takes about half a minute and involves hardly any undressing. Doctors will often take the opportunity quickly to check the pressure during a visit to the surgery for some other reason.

Who has hypertension?

Anybody can have it. No particular group seems to be specially vulnerable, but blacks get it more often than whites. It is equally common in men and women. Blood pressure tends to increase with age so hypertension is commoner in older people. But this does not mean that raised pressure in older people should be regarded as harmless. Up to the age of 65 years the extra risk for a particular pressure seems to be similar whether the subject is 30 or 60 years old. Over 65 the picture is less clear, largely because few studies have been carried out. Doctors are cautious about treating the elderly without symptoms. Some evidence suggests that women in their 70s and 80s are more tolerant of an elevated pressure.

My doctor told me that my blood pressure was 160/105, but he did not start any treatment. Why?

Treatment of hypertension implies a lifelong commitment. Once the pressure has been reduced it is difficult to assess whether therapy is needed. An individual's blood pressure varies quite markedly and may be highest during the mild anxiety of a medical consultation. Unless there is already clear evidence of damage due to hypertension, several blood pressure measurements will be necessary to get the true picture. In this example, the doctor may have had lower readings in the past, or he may have decided just to repeat the measurement at the next opportunity.

Another possible explanation is that all subject with hypertension do not require treatment. In particular, elderly people find the tablets difficult to take for years and the benefits of treatment in this age group are less certain. If other medical problems are present, hypertension may be best left undisturbed while the major event is dealt with. Some people find regular tablet taking impossible and treatment of their raised pressure may be unrealistic. Like so many aspects of medicine, hard and fast rules cannot be applied and it is up to the doctor and his patient to arrive at the best decision.

Can we really justify the cost and inconvenience of treating all these people with symptomless hypertension?

If the current studies do show that even mild hypertension should be treated, the implications are rather frightening. Some of these mild hypertensives will be able to control the pressure by non-drug means (p.90) but most will not. Population studies show that 30-40 percent of people have either a diastolic pressure above 90 millimetres of\mercury,\or a systolic pressure\above 140 millimetres (or both). The current studies may show that they need treatment. Some will not require it for a variety of reasons, but we still might end up with a quarter of the whole population on drugs for high blood pressure. In most the treatment would continue for ever.

The cost and effort of treating all these people would be considerable. But the cost and effort of treating a stroke or heart failure is much larger. If clear evidence is obtained that mildly raised pressure should be lowered to prevent complications and that the drugs can be readily tolerated, the large numbers will have to be treated. Hopefully a sub-group of people particularly at risk will be identified in the future. Treatment could then be concentrated on this group. But as yet, a high-risk category of mildly hypertensive individuals has not been found.

Blood lipids

Blood fats, or more correctly blood lipids, have fascinated scientists and doctors for years. In spite of three decades of intensive research by these experts, the lipids' precise role and importance in the genesis of coronary artery disease remain controversial. The field has tended to attract enthusiasts who sometimes let their hopes leap ahead of their facts. The resulting disagreements can be embarrassing. We will try to find a route through this minefield, maintaining a distinction between what may be true and what has been shown to be true. At the outset it is important to remember that dietary fats and blood fats are not interchangeable concepts. Food intake certainly influences the blood lipids but it is not the sole determinant.

What are the blood lipids?

The two imporant blood lipids are cholesterol and trglyceride. Lipids do not circulate freely in the blood but are incorporated in complexes with protein and phospholipids known as lipoproteins. The lipoproteins are carriers of the cholesterol and triglyceride. Their classification is based on their physical properties. Four broad categories are described:

Chylomicrons

Chylomicrons consist mostly of triglyceride absorbed from dietary fat in the intestines. Normally, they disappear after 12 hours of fasting.

Very low density lipoproteins (VLDL)

The lipid in these complexes is mostly triglyceride released from the liver. The concentration of VLDL is increased by obesity. Their association with heart disease is not strong.

Low density lipoproteins (LDL)

These lipoproteins contain a high concentration of cholesterol and are the most directly associated with coronary artery disease.

High density lipoproteins (HDL)

Cholesterol is also the main lipid in HDL but its cardiac effects are opposite to LDL. A raised concentration of HDL is associated with *less* heart disease.

For a single subject the composition of the blood lipids or lipoproteins can be expressed in a number of ways. The blood is always taken after a 12 hour fast to prevent any distortion by a recent meal. The simplest determination is to break up the lipoproteins and meaure the total concentrations of both cholesterol and triglyceride. A total cholesterol level has often been used as a measure of blood lipids for experimental studies of risk factors.

A more difficult, but more helpful, method is to determine the lipoprotein concentrations. This is done by electrophoresis — a technique that uses the differing densities and electrical charges of the lipoproteins for separation. Fredrickson and colleagues proposed a classification for familial hyperlipidaemias, that is inherited forms of raised blood lipids. The classification was quickly extended to all hyperlipidaemias; in any case, hereditary factors are important in the more severe examples. Fredrickson's classification divides into five types, with one subdivided:

Type 1 Excess chylomicrons, no increased risk of heart disease
Type 2a Raised LDL, increased risk of coronary artery disease.
Type 2b Raised LDL and VLDL, increased risk of coronary
   artery disease.

Type 3 Essentially familial pattern with lipoprotein appearing as a broad band on electrophoresis, increased risk of coronary artery disease.

Type 4 Increased VLDL, sometimes associated with diabetes. May have an increased risk of coronary artery disease.

Type 5   Excess chylomicrons and VLDL, no increased risk of heart disease.

This classification is cumbersome for routine work. Another method, which may have more practical importance, is to measure the cholesterol in the other high density lipoproteins and the cholesterol in the other lipoproteins. This seems to give us the best guide to the risk of future heart disease because, as discussed later, HDL cholesterol seems to have some protective effect while the other cholesterol is associated with heart disease.

Is an elevated cholesterol level associated with coronary artery disease?

Yes, the association is strong. Countries with an above average blood cholesterol level tend to have more deaths from coronary artery disease than those with a lower level. Within one country, people with raised concentrations of cholesterol are more liable to develop the diseases. In Britain a man with a blood cholesterol level of 8 mMol/litre (300 mg/dl) has three times the risk of dying from heart disease than a man with a blood cholesterol level of 4 mMol/1 (150 mg/dl).

But an elevated blood cholesterol is not associated with a greater chance of heart disease in everybody. If the extra cholesterol is in the HDL form, it is protective and can reduce the chances of myocardial infarction. Unfortunately, in most people the extra cholesterol is in the LDL form. This is why, in general, a raised concentration is associated with an increased risk of coronary artery disease.

Why is a raised blood cholesterol associated with heart disease?

This is a difficult question to answer. Atherosclerosis is a human problem. Experimental animals do not get it, which means that we cannot answer the question by straightforward laboratory work. A sort of arterial disease can be induced in experimental animals be feeding them on a very abnormal diet with a high concentration of fat. But many experts feel that this arterial damage is not the same as atherosclerosis.

Cholesterol is present in the atherosclerotic arterial wall. One suggstion is that the uptake of cholesterol by the arterial wall is normally balanced by a similar rate of release back into the blood. If this two-way balance is disturbed, perhaps by a higher concentration of cholesterol in the blood, then atherosclerosis may be the result as the cholesterol accumulates in the wall. Another possibility is that certain lipoproteins, which contain cholesterol, may stimulate the cells of the arterial wall to divide prematurely. This could disorganize the basic wall structure and promote atherosclerosis. All these mechanisms are still speculative at present.

Why is HDL cholesterol protective?

One suggestion is that these lipoproteins are transporting cholesterol away from the arterial wall. The reduction in the wall cholesterol could be responsible for a reduced amount of atherosclerosis, but this is unproven.

What causes raised lipids in the blood?

In a few people is is an inherited abnormality. The lipids are markedly abnormal and may collect in patches under the skin. Members of some affected families can develop coronary artery disease at a very young age.

But these familial abnormalities are rare. For most people a modest elevation in the fat levels has no particular cause. Like hypertension we are dealing with a continuous range of values, some of which are associated with heart disease and we call them abnormal. No sharp division exists between normal and abnormal values. It follows from this that the division is somewhat arbitrary. The upper limit for a normal cholesterol is often around 7 mMol/1 (270 mg/dl) and for triglyceride is 2 mMol/1 (180 mg/dl). But rather different figures will often be quoted.

Do changes in blood lipids reduce the risk of developing coronary artery disease?

This is one of the key questions in the prevention of heart disease.

Opinions differ quite markedly. To repeat a theme of this chapter, demonstrating an association between raised lipids and coronary artery disease is not the same as being able to prevent heart disease by lowering the lipids.

The best way of establishing this would be to reduce the lipids in a group of people and then see whether they had less heart trouble compared to an otherwise identical group with unchanged lipids. But such investigations are very difficult. The 'incubation period' for coronary artery disease is ten years or more, so prolonged studies are needed. Sustaining any changes for many years is very hard for some people. Also large alterations in blood lipid levels are difficult to achieve. Smokers can reduce their cigarette usage by 100 per cent — they stop smoking. But most individuals with raised lipids find a cholesterol reduction of more than 20 per cent very hard to achieve. An additional complication is that the protective effects of HDL cholesterol have only been appreciated in the last few years. In some people a reduction in the HDL cholesterol could negate any benefits from lowering total cholesterol. All but the most recent studies fail to make any allowances for this.

No study by itself proves unequivocably that changing blood lipids reduces the risk of heart disease, though some evidence supports this conclusion. A prolonged investigation in a Finnish mental hospital involved reducing the blood cholesterol in half the patients with a low animal fat diet. A modest reduction in heart disease was demonstrated but the design of the trial, and therefore its scientific validity, have been questioned.

Most recent studies aimed at reducing several risk factors. The subjects are exhorted to stop smoking and take more exercise as well as reducing their blood lipids. Work in Scandinavia has suggested that the risk of coronary artery disease can be reduced by this multifactorial approach. Reviewing the results in detail, the reduction in lipids seems important but the change in other risk factors might also be a major influence. One problem of this type of study is that the group of men, who are just kept under observation for comparison, receive advice about heart disease prevention from other sources and start to lead a healthier life. An enormous American study on prevention recently reported an inconclusive result, possibly because the 'control' group spontaneously corrected some of their risk factors. But another American study did show a reduction in mortality as a result of blood lipid modification, though the subjects had to take an unpleasant drug for several years to achieve it.

At the moment some experts will preach vehemently that reducing blood lipids is the key to the 20th century epidemic of coronary artery disease. Other will take the opposite view and say that the benefits of adjusting the lipids are very marginal and not worth the effort. Most doctors are somewhere in between. They feel that the benefits of reducing lipids have not yet been completely proved but at this time it seems a reasonable conclusion. They would conclude that a general reduction in the amount of animal fat in the diet is desirable but that most individuals should not worry unduly about the precise level of their blood cholesterol.

Do changes in blood lipids reduce the risk of a recurrence of coronary artery disease?

So far, we have considered whether altering the lipids will prevent the development of heart disease in a previously healthy person. But should a patient who already has angina or a myocardial infarction attempt to change these fats to avoid further trouble? Once again, experts differ on this question.

Many doctors feel that, once the coronary artery atherosclerosis has formed, attempting to correct lipid abnormalities will achieve little. An exception to this would be the occasional patient with a severe, familial, lipid abnormality who might benefit from such treatment. These patients are uncommon. Unlike the association with the development of coronary artery disease, the cholesterol concentration in the blood seems to have little bearing on the risk of recurrence of heart disease. Nevertheless doctors will often measure the blood fats, particularly in younger patients. One of the aims is to identify subjects with very high levels so that their close relatives can be screened.

Other doctors agree that lifelong prevention is better than closing the stable door once the horse has bolted. But they say that every possible effort should be made in the hope that a few patients might benefit. Certainly there seems little harm in adopting some of the simple dietary measures for improving

lipids as described later in this section. More controversy
as to whether drug therapy is justified for this purpose.
doctors would say not in the majority of cases, but
exceptions can be found.

How can blood lipids be improved?

Until recently this meant just a reduction of a raised cholesterol
or triglyceride concentration. But now that the protective effects
of HDL cholesterol have been recognized, an increase in this
class of lipoproteins would be desirable.

A change in the diet is the commonest method of adjusting the
blood lipids. Unfortunately food intake is only one of several
influences on the body's cholesterol and triglyceride concentrations. A diet can modify lipids to some extent, but unless the food
consumption has been grossly abnormal beforehand the changes
may not be great.

The basic principle of the diet is to reduce the amount of
animal fat eaten, remembering that milk, milk products, and egg
yolks are also prime sources. Much of animal fat is 'saturated'.
This is a chemical term referring to the linkage between carbon
atoms in the fat molecule. Vegetable fats are rather more
'unsaturated' (or 'polyunsaturated') as the carbon atoms have
'spare' linkages. In general saturated fat is bad for the heart
while polyunsaturated fat is much better. The overall strategy is
to reduce the total fat intake by substituting carbohydrates and
to have as much as possible of the remaining fats in the
polyunsaturated form.

In practice the quantity of beef, pork, and lamb in the diet
should be reduced and replaced by vegetables, fish, and chicken.
Fat should be trimmed off meat and the 'crackling' avoided. The
quantity of fat mixed in with meat fibres is high enough even with
the fat removed from the edges. Chicken is a good alternative to
meat, as most of the fat is in the skin. Other poultry such as duck
has more fat in the flesh and may be less satisfactory. Milk and
cheese intake should be reduced and the amount of cream
consumed kept to a minimum. Cream can appear in a number of
disguises such as chocolate, mayonnaise, and some ice cream.
'Low-cholesterol' margarines can replace butter, particularly in
cooking.

The methods of cooking are also important. Grilling or roasting with the fat being allowed to drain away are the best methods. Any frying should be done in a vegetable oil which is high in poly-unsaturated fat such as sunflower oil, corn oil, or soya bean oil. Non-specific 'vegetable oil' could contain anything. Egg whites can be used freely, but egg yolks have a high cholesterol content and should not be eaten too often.

Fruit and vegetables can be eaten without restriction. A few, such as coconuts, have a lot of saturated fats, but none of these is liable to be consumed in a significant amount. With the exception of walnuts, nuts have a high concentration of the wrong fats and should not be eaten in large quantities.

This type of 'cholesterol-reducing' diet is familiar to many people. But there are two common misconceptions. One is to confuse 'weight-reducing' with 'cholesterol reducing'. Some foods, such as most vegetables are suitable for both purposes. Others, such as low-cholesterol margarines, have just as many calories as the foods they replace (butter, in this case). The other misconception is to assume that all fats of non-animal origin are satisfactory. Coconut oil with its saturated fats has already been mentioned. In ordinary hard margarines some of the fat has been treated to convert unsaturated linkages to the saturated form. This hardens the margarine so that it can be packed like butter, but it also means that these margarines are not a good substitute for butter. In any case a 'cholesterol-reducing' diet should involve a reduction in the total fat intake, not just a switch from animal fats to vegetable fats.

If diet fails to achieve a satisfactory reduction in the cholesterol and triglyceride should drugs be used?

Until the late 1970s drug therapy was quite popular as an addition to adjusting food intake. It did not solve everybody's lipid problems but at least the tablets were felt to be fairly harmless. The most popular drug was clofibrate (Atromid-S). A large trial was started in Britain and two other European countries to see whether clofibrate treatment was effective in preventing heart disease. In 1978 the results were reported The incidence of coronary artery disease was indeed less amongst the men treated with clofibrate compared to those untreated; but it was a big surprise to find that the treated men had *more* deaths overall. The extra deaths were not due to any one cause. In other words clofibrate seemed to offer some protection against coronary artery disease, but it had other effects which are associated with an increased risk of death from non-cardiac disease. These effects are still uncertain.

The result of the clofibrate trial has cast a shadow over the drug treatment of raised lipids. Clofibrate is now reserved for severe cases which do not respond to other means. Other drugs can be prescribed, but none has been investigated as extensively as clofibrate. So although these newer drugs seem safer, doctors are reluctant to use them unless the need is clear.

Although an increase in the HDL cholesterol would be beneficial it is not easy to achieve. A low animal fat diet or cholesterol-lowering drugs will tend to reduce the HDL cholesterol along with other cholesterol. Correction of obesity usually increases HDL cholesterol without affecting other cholesterol adversely. Some studies, but not all, have shown that regular exercise has the same beneficial result. Further information on this important topic should soon be available.

Fortunately, regular exercise and maintenance of a satisfactory weight can already be recommended for other reasons.

Could adjusting the blood lipids be harmful?

The clofibrate trial forced doctors to look at this question rather more seriously than they did in the past. It had often been assumed that modest changes in the lipids might not do much good, but at least they did not do any harm. Now we are not quite so sure. Cholesterol-lowering regimes tend to promote the formation of gall stones which are often painful and occasionally are the cause of a major illness. A more serious charge is that the regimes are associated with an increased incidence of bowel cancer. So far this has not been established. It would seem very unlikely that a diet could produce a sufficient effect. Drug therapy is a more plausible cause, but it has not been implicated convincingly. It is another reminder for doctors only to prescribe the drugs when the necessity is clear.

Exercise

The need for regular exercise in the prevention of heart disease is another controversial point. It makes you feel better, but does it reduce the risk of heart disease?

Is lack of exercise associated with coronary artery disease?

It probably is, but the evidence is not clearcut. Well-motivated people who exert themselves frequently do seem to have less heart disease. But the same individuals will also usually be non-smokers and pay attention to their diet and weight. Unskilled manual workers who exert themselves in the course of their jobs and do not worry about risk factors are not often included in this type of study as they work long hours and cannot get time off for special clinics. In general, men who exercise seem to get less heart disease, though the mechanism is uncertain.

Is lack of exercise a cause of coronary artery disease?

Regular exercise will enable the heart to function more efficiently. The heart can work harder so that the man or woman will be able to do more and feel better as a result. Exercise will certainly promote heath in the general sense of the word. But this is not the same as preventing heart disease. Atherosclerosis could be developing in the coronary arteries in spite of an improvement in the efficiency of the heart muscle.

Some evidence is available to show that exercise can diminish the chance of developing heart disease. But, as so often happens in the field of prevention, the evidence is not conclusive. American studies have shown the benefits of exercise in reducing the incidence of coronary artery disease; but it has to be done often — three times a week or more. Frequency may be more important than the severity of exertion. The implication is that exercise as part of the daily routine (such as cycling to work) is better than the occasional session (a game of squash, for example). At the moment, exercise can be recommended as part of the strategy to prevent heart disease but more information is needed.

Is exercise beneficial once coronary artery disease has appeared?

This question has already been answered in Chapter 4. Briefly, rest is part of the initial treatment of myocardial infarction or crescendo angina, but it should not be prolonged unduly. Once the acute phase is over exercise will improve the efficiency of the

197

heart and enable the patient to do more. It could go some way to preventing a recurrence.

Could exercise be harmful?

Earlier in this century many medical treatments involved a period of rest and, in a vague manner, rest was felt to be good for everybody. This may have been a reflection of the necessity then for many men and women to work long hours in physically exhausting jobs. Perhaps the recent emphasis on the benefits of exercise has been sparked off by the widespread adoption of sedentary employment. As far as we can tell exercise does no harm in the majority of people. The main exception is those individuals who already have severe or unstable heart disease: exercise could precipitate further damage. People over 45 years old should ask their doctor's advice before indulging in severe exertion which is unfamiliar to them. At any age a new activity should be started gradually.

Although major harmful effects are very rare, minor ailments are more common. A wide variety of muscular aches and pains can be induced, especially soon after starting. They will settle but not without some soreness for a time.

Doctors have speculated whether really severe exercise sustained for many years could damage the heart. The hearts of top-class marathon runners enlarge significantly to cope with the increased physical demands and they also beat slowly at rest. Marathon runners can still get coronary artery disease; but no evidence has been found of an increased risk of any form of heart disease compared to non-runners. The available information suggests that a heart is not damaged by this type of running even though it becomes enlarged.

How much exercise should be undertaken?

This will depend on a person's age, general state of health, and degree of training. A general rule is that a fresh activity should be started gradually. If you restart cycling after a gap of several years, just going up one steep hill may be enough on the first day; this can be progressively extended to rides of many miles. You should aim to do enough exercise to make yourself a little breathless three times a week. The pulse rate is a good guide to the amount of work the heart is doing. To avoid excessive exertion the rate per minute should not exceed 190 minus your age in years. The body will soon become fitter, allowing the severity of exercise to be increased. A pre-existing medical condition should be assessed by a doctor before starting.

The best form of exercise will vary. Most people think of jogging in this context. This can be an enjoyable form of exertion and mental relaxation which can be done almost anywhere, with or without companions. But some find it extremely boring and may prefer active sports. Running or cycling to work can save money and, in big cities, time. Even just avoiding the lift and walking quickly up several flights of stairs instead is useful. For older people golf or a brisk walk can provide the necessary exertion. Exercise that involves movement is better for the heart than heaving or pushing activities such as weightlifting or digging the garden. But above all, try and make it fun. Regardless of the original intentions, a tedious activity will be stopped eventually.

Stress

As we have already seen in Chapter 4, stress is difficult to define and almost impossible to measure. One man's stress is another's interesting challenge. Dimly, two forms of stress can be recognized. One is the chronic form produced by long-lasting problems such as an unhappy marriage, troublesome children, or difficulty in managing a job. The other is an acute reaction to an unplanned event such as an accident, being sacked from a job or a heated argument.

Is chronic stress a cause of heart disease?

Popular mythology clings to the belief that the person most vulnerable to a myocardial infarction is a high-powered executive who is under constant stress of decision making and meeting deadlines. Some doctors have cultivated this idea, perhaps because such executives are a good source of private practice. Unfortunately, it is not true, at least not for the last 30 years. In the first half of this century managers and professional men did seem to develop coronary artery disease more often than unskilled workers, but since about 1950 the reverse has been true. For example, a study of British civil servants showed that the unskilled office workers developed more coronary artery disease than the top grade civil servants. American studies in large corporations have also shown that the more senior the executive, the less vulnerable he is to heart disease. Of course, this does not prove that any stress of decision making is beneficial. The distribution of risk factors is important; for example, the unskilled workers tend to smoke more.

So the harmful effects of chronic stress have been exaggerated. Indeed it is possible that chronic stress is irrelevant to heart disease, but we cannot say this for certain as this type of stress is not amenable to measurement. The talented, ambitious executive may be under less stress in his job than a frustrated worker in a boring job with insufficient money for his family's needs. Experts have speculated whether the stress of unemployment could be a cause of heart disease. So far the evidence is equivocal and any conclusions may partly reflect the political belief of the expert. No form of chronic stress has been shown to have a major role in the genesis of coronary artery disease, but a minor effect cannot be ruled out. The difficulties of measuring stress not only make it hard to prove a relationship, but they also hamper efforts to exclude it as a cause of heart disease.

Could acute stress be harmful?

Acute stress is easier to investigate than the chronic form. The unplanned stressful event produces measurable effects on the body in the form of the so-called 'fight or flight reaction'. This protective mechanism, which is left over from prehistoric times, involves an increase in the heart rate, improved alertness, and a shift in some of the blood circulation to the muscles from other organs. The body is then better equipped to fight the aggressor or run away, as appropriate. This response is mediated by parts of the nervous system and also by circulating messenger chemicals (hormones) known as catecholamines. The catecholamines can be measured in the blood or urine.

This acute reaction to stress does no harm to a healthy person. But the effects on a diseased heart can be more troublesome. The reaction stimulates the heart, increasing its oxygen requirements. This can produce an attack of angina in a vulnerable subject with narrowed coronary arteries. Occasionally, acute stress may be the precipitating event for a myocardial infarction. But it is not the main cause and such an infarction would have happened anyway at some time.

The nerve stimulation and catecholamine release speed up the heart in acute stress and can also make diseased ventricular muscle more electrically excitable. Abnormal heart rhythms, such as ventricular tachycardia or even fibrillation (p.138) can then be started more easily. These abnormal rhythms are commoner immediately after a myocardial infarction, so acute stress is particularly harmful at this time. In addition ventricular fibrillation is the commonest cause of sudden cardiac death (p.75) outside hospital. Could acute stress be involved? Animal work suggests that it may be a factor and it has been implicated as one possible cause of sudden cardiac death amongst people who already are at risk due to certain forms of coronary artery disease.

The precise importance of acute stress is still uncertain, but it does have some role in the genesis of complications amongst people who already have coronary artery disease. So good advice to patients with this form of heart trouble is to 'keep cool and count to ten'. Some of this type of stress cannot be avoided if life is going to be worth living, but it should be kept to a minimum in patients with heart disease. They should try to be relaxed in response to stressful events. In any case, dealing with a problem calmly and rationally can be much more effective than 'blowing your top'.

Will a change of job to avoid stress be beneficial?

Anybody who finds his job physically or mentally exhausting can be advised to change it in order to regain a sense of well being. But no evidence exists to prove that changing a job will prevent the development of heart disease. No occupation is associated with a particular risk of coronary artery atherosclerosis. Once heart disease is present, a change to a less demanding job may be worth while to improve the quality of life and perhaps to avoid too much acute stress. But most patients with heart disease do not need to change jobs.

Personality

The influence of personality on the development of heart disease is a popular topic. Technical terms like type A and type B personalities are used widely. The division into these two groups is simple — perhaps too simple. Personality is often linked to other potential risk factors. In particular, this section overlaps with the previous one as a person's response to a stressful event is largely conditioned by his or her personality.

What are type A and type B personalities?

The concept of these two classes was formulated in America over 20 years ago. People with type A personalities are determined and aggressive. They are aware of deadlines and can concentrate on a particular activity to the exclusion of everything else. Type B people are more relaxed and able to let life drift by, savouring the good things in it. Of course, this represents the opposite poles of the type A/Type B personality spectrum. Many people are somewhere in between.

Why is personality important?

Several studies have shown that men or women with type A personalities have a greater chance of developing coronary artery disease than those with type B. The reason for this is uncertain. Risk factors such as smoking and diet are not distributed evenly between the two groups, but their variation is not enough to explain the different incidence of heart disease amongst the two personality types. Another possibility is that type A personality is associated with a more marked reaction to acute stress.

Whether these personality differences have any practical importance is doubtful. Personalities cannot be altered, though in theory behaviour patterns can be. But at the moment there is no evidence that altering behaviour will help. Up to 45 per cent of an unselected population have a type A personality, so identifying people with this characteristic will do little to delineate those at particularly high risk of getting heart disease. Determining personality is about as helpful in preventing heart disease as determining sex. Type A personalities and men both have a higher incidence of trouble compared to type Bs and women, but little or nothing can be done to change these factors.

Obesity

Fat people are more vulnerable to coronary artery disease than thin people. They are also more prone to diabetes, respiratory problems, muscular and joint disorders, and other disabilities. The link with coronary artery disease is not straightforward. Obesity is associated with other risk factors such as hypertension, raised blood lipids, diabetes, and lack of exercise. Fat people are more likely to exhibit these factors than thin people. Recent work suggests that the apparent association of obesity with heart disease may be due to these other factors. Obesity is important, but its deleterious effects on the heart seem to be indirect.

Whatever the precise mechanisms, weight reduction plays a major role in the prevention and control of heart disease. Like smoking, but unlike blood lipids, weight can be changed drastically with a big improvement in health. Successful dieters look and feel better, in addition to the long-term benefits of reducing their risk of heart disease. An inspection of the local newspaper will show very few fat citizens photographed at their ninetieth or hundredth birthday parties; they are almost all thin.

What is the best way to lose weight?

Nobody should be short of advice on how to lose weight. Magazines are full of articles and books flow from the publishers in a torrent. Unfortunately none can avoid the central issue; the only way to lose a significant amount of weight is to eat fewer calories. Increased exercise can augment this as long as the resulting appetite improvement can be controlled. Losing weight takes time. The first few pounds come off easily, but after that it is slow going. Several months are required for a significant reduction and considerable effort is needed.

The best weight reducing diet is the one that works. Many people can manage on a standard diet which involves a general reduction in foods rich in fats and carbohydrates. Fatty foods particularly should be kept to a minimum as fat has twice as many calories as the same weight of carbohydrates. Skilful advertising by the dairy industry has reinforced the belief that milk, and milk products such as cheese, butter and cream, are healthy. But within a balanced diet no one food has particular merit. When dieting, more will be achieved by reducing the intake of these fatty products than by cutting back on a few potatoes. A reduction in animal fat intake has already been recommended in the section on blood lipids earlier in this chapter. An ordinary low-fat diet will produce two desirable effects — weight reduction and blood lipid reduction. With carbohydrates the quantities matter, not the type of carbohydrate. Pound for pound, the carbohydrates, such as bread, potatoes, cakes, and sugar, have a similar number of calories. Remember that alcoholic drinks, especially beer, also contain a significant number of calories.

Some dieters find 'freakish' regimes easier. These diets usually involve eating large quantities of one food while reducing the amount of everything else. The single food proves very boring and the large quantities diminish, reducing the total amount eaten. Such diets can be satisfactory for a few weeks but they are difficult to sustain for the necessary months. Taken to extremes they could lead to malnutrition after a few weeks, but this seems to happen rarely.

Why are some people apparently unable to lose weight?

Some dieters, especially middle-aged women, often complain that they have tried everything without success. Losing weight is a matter of making the calorie intake less than the calorie requirements. So the correct intake is partly determined by the amount of physical exertion a person performs. But even allowing for this calorie requirements vary markedly. Some people seem to utilize their food efficiently and so need fewer calories. With identical diets and degree of physical exertion, one person can gain weight and another lose it.

But everybody has a level of consumption below which they lose weight. When food is in short supply, as in World War Two concentration camps, nobody is fat. This is not to deny that some unfortunate people deal with their food very efficiently and only require a modest intake. Such subjects will always have difficulty in controlling their weight, but it can be done. In practice food intake is often greater than is appreciated. Detailed observations of women who 'cannot lose weight' have shown that the subjects may inadvertently eat much more than they think. Few, if any, people will not shed weight on a genuine 1,000 calories diet sustained for several weeks.

If the response to dieting is poor, it is easy to become disheartened. But the effort has not been wasted; without the diet weight would probably have gone up. A few days' increase can take months of effort to remove; so prevention is always worth while. The diet will also accustom the body to a reduced intake, making later dieting easier.

Diabetes

The individual cells of the organs get much of their energy supplies in the form of glucose. The uptake of glucose from the blood into the cells is under the control of insulin secreted by the body's own pancreas. In diabetes this insulin is in short supply with the result that the glucose concentration rises in the blood and falls in the cells. Some of the extra glucose in the blood finds its way into the urine. Testing for glucose (loosely described as 'sugar') in the urine is a simple method for detecting diabetes.

Depriving the cells of some of their energy supply has widespread effects in the body. The particular relevance to this chapter is that diabetes encourages the formation of coronary artery atherosclerosis. Any degree of diabetes seems to be associated with an increased incidence of heart disease. So prevention of diabetes could reduce the risk of heart disease. In younger patients the shortage of insulin is not preventable, but in some older subjects it is secondary to obesity. This is an additional reason to control weight.

At one time it was hoped that the successful treatment of diabetes with insulin injections, tablets, or a diet alone would help to prevent heart disease. Unfortunately correct treatment has not been shown to reduce the cardiac risk. Several explanations can be put forward. The coronary arteries may already be damaged before the diabetes is discovered. Another possibility is that treatment does not mimic satisfactorily the subtle glucose adjustments achieved by natural insulin from a healthy pancreas. A third suggestion is that the atherosclerosis is not simply due to a shortage of glucose in the cells; the true mechanism could be more complex and not correctable by current methods of treatment.

One American study suggested that certain tablets used in the treatment of diabetes could increase the chances of developing heart disease. The implication was that diabetics should all be using insulin injections rather than tablets. But these findings have not been generally accepted in Britain; other studies have failed to show the same effect. At the moment there is no reason to avoid tablet therapy for diabetes if it is effective.

Hypothyrodism

An underactive thyroid gland (hypothyroidism) is associated with an increased risk of developing coronary artery disease. The deficiency of the thyroid hormone produces marked changes in blood lipids, especially a rise in the LDL cholesterol (p.189). These changes will promote the formation of atherosclerosis.

The relevance of this to the prevention of heart trouble is limited. Hypothyroidism is a fairly uncommon disorder and potential victims cannot be predicted in advance. However, once the disease has become apparent, treatment may halt the progression of the coronary atherosclerosis. Newborn babies can be screened to detect an underactive thyroid gland but there are no plans to extend this to adults.

Gout

For some reason gout is often regarded as a joke. Sufferers know it as a very painful inflammation of a joint, often one in the foot. It is caused by an excess of uric acid in the blood which is then deposited in the joint to produce the inflammation. Uric acid is one of the body's waste products. It is normally removed by the kidneys, but in gout the kidneys cannot remove it fast enough.

A raised uric acid concentration in the blood is also mildly associated with an increased risk of coronary artery disease. Not all studies have demonstrated this, but many have. The consensus view is that a raised uric acid concentration is probably a risk factor, though its cardiac effects may be very mild. Or to put it the other way round, most people with gout do not have heart trouble. The true importance of a raised uric acid level is undecided. This is more than an academic question because, unlike many risk factors, the blood uric acid concentration can be reduced quite sharply by drug therapy. Many people have a moderate elevation of uric acid concentration without any gout. At the moment long-term drug therapy cannot be recommended for them, but this may change.

Water softness

A soft water supply is associated with a locally increased risk of coronary artery disease. This surprising finding has been confirmed in different countries though not every survey has shown it.

As yet, the reason for this association is uncertain. It could be a chance finding reflecting some other linked risk factor but this factor has not yet been found. At least one study has indicated that the overall incidence of coronary artery disease may not differ much between hard and soft water areas, but that sudden cardiac deaths (p.74) are commoner with a soft water supply. If this is confirmed it means that the softness has little to do with the formation of atherosclerosis but is more related to the creation of fatal ventricular rhythm disturbances, such as ventricular fibrillation (p.75), in people with pre-existing heart disease.

Water hardness is produced by an increased mineral content. But the mineral responsible will vary from one hard water supply to another. Attempts to determine the minerals associated with a decreased risk of heart trouble have not proved conclusive. Until the specific agents have been found, no advice can be given about possible additions to the water supply. But household water softeners might be harmful, even if they do make the washing easier.

Alcohol

Excessive alcohol is certainly harmful to health in a variety of ways. Alcoholism, which can be defined as dependency on alcohol, is very destructive for self-esteem, family relationships, and job prospects. Over the years cirrhosis of the liver leads to eventual liver failure. In a few people alcohol has direct toxic effects on the heart. The muscle is poisoned and heart failure follows. Large quantities of alcohol are needed for this effect — perhaps eight pints of beer a day or its equivalent. An interesting recent finding is that more moderate alcohol consumption is associated with an increased chance of developing hypertension. As described earlier, the raised pressure will augment the risk of getting heart disease.

What about the effects of moderate 'social' drinking?

Interestingly some recent surveys suggest that a modest alcohol intake could protect against coronary artery disease. The emphasis is on 'modest'. Using the convention that the alcohol contents of a standard tot of spirits, a glass of wine or sherry, and half a pint of beer are all similar and can be referred to as one drink, people who have one or two drinks a day seem to show less heart disease than those who take none or more than two drinks a day. Certainly a small daily amount of alcohol does not seen to harm the heart. But remember that the quantities are small; we are talking about pub measures, not the amount a person might pour into his own glass.

How could the alcohol be beneficial?

Alcohol is a mild vasodilator, that is it increases the size of the arteries slightly. In the presence of some coronary artery athero-sclerosis a mild dilatation might be just enough to ward off angina or to avoid a myocardial infarction. Another possibility is the influence of alcohol in increasing the HDL cholesterol (p.189). At the moment only speculation is possible.

Coffee

One American survey has shown that heavy coffee drinkers seem more liable to heart disease than non-coffee drinkers. But other studies have failed to confirm this and at the moment coffee drinking is not regarded as a risk factor. As most of the work has been done in the United States tea drinking has not received any attention, but nothing suggests that it has any role in creating heart disease.

A few people who already have heart disease may notice adverse effects from drinking coffee. Caffeine, the main stimulant in coffee, can have a direct action on the heart in an occasional patient. The ventricular muscle is rendered more excitable by the caffeine. This encourages the formation of extra beats —ventricular ectopic beats (p.139). The patient may not be aware of them or he may notice an irregular palpitation. In an extreme case the heart may be stimulated into an abnormal, fast rhythm —ventricular tachycardia (p.138). These effects can be avoided in the few susceptible patients by reducing the amount of coffee drunk or by switching to a decaffeinated brand.

Dietary fibre

Over the last few years interest in dietary fibre has grown. Fibre is the indigestible portion of plant cells in the diet ('roughage'); it passes through the intestine and into the motions without being absorbed by the body. Fibre has been shown to have a role in the prevention and treatment of many diseases, especially those involving the bowel. A suggestion has been made that increased dietary fibre may reduce the incidence of coronary artery disease. Populations with a large intake of fibre, mainly those in underdeveloped countries, have a low risk of heart disease. But they also have a low incidence of known cardiac risk factors. Increasing the amount of fibre in the food can have a beneficial effect on the blood lipids, but we do not know whether this is followed by less coronary atherosclerosis. At the moment the potential cardiac benefits of dietary fibre must be regarded as unproven. More information should emerge soon.

Dietary sugar

In general usage sugar refers to one carbohydrate with the biochemical name of sucrose. But to biochemists sugars are a wide range of carbohydrates of which sucrose is an example. The 'sugar' in the urine of untreated diabetics is glucose not sucrose. Here we are referring to sugar in the sense of meaning just sucrose.

As described earlier, coronary artery disease is a disease of civilization, that is Western civilization. And one of the most noticeable features of the Western 'civilized' diet is the amount of refined sugar consumed. Sugar does not occur naturally in a pure form. It has to be extracted from sugarcane or sugarbeet. So the diet of primitive people does not contain it. The hypothesis has been advanced that dietary sugar is associated with the risk of developing heart disease.

Some evidence exists that sugar consumption is related to heart disease, though it has not been universally accepted. Sugar in large quantities has other adverse effects such as weight gain or encouraging diabetes, so a prudent diet will avoid excessive consumption anyway. Leaving most food unsweetened would seem to be desirable.

Dietary salt

Patients with coronary artery disease are sometimes recommended to reduce the amount of salt in their food. The purpose of this is to keep their blood pressures at a normal level. As mentioned on page 90 dietary salt has a role in the creation of hypertension. Patients with heart disease should not allow their blood pressures to creep up.

A reduction in the salt intake of people without any heart disease should reduce the overall incidence of hypertension. This would have a secondary effect of preventing some cases of coronary artery disease. But at present dietary salt is not regarded as a direct risk factor.

Oral contraceptives

Oral contraceptives are very safe and reliable. They are safer than most other tablets and also safer than the pregnancy they are designed to prevent. But unlike other drugs which are used to treat illnesses, oral contraceptives are given to healthy women. For this reason particularly high standards of safety are required.

The chemical effects of oral contraceptives are detectable throughout the body. Their relevance to heart disease is that they encourage blood clotting to a slight extent. Surveys have shown that some women on the drugs have an increased risk of developing a myocardial infarction. Women over 35, especially if they are smokers, and those who have been taking the tablets for many years have been identified as being vulnerable.

The increased risk of heart disease should be kept in perspective. A myocardial infarction is very rare in a woman under 40 years old and taking the oral contraceptives only increases the risk a little. Nevertheless, it is now recommended that women over 35 years old should consider alternative methods, particularly if they are also smokers. Remaining on the tablets continously from teenage to 35 years old is also best avoided. These suggestions may not be appropriate to every woman. If there is no reasonable alternative method of preventing an unwanted pregnancy, the mild increase in risk may be acceptable.

Conclusion

In this chapter many of the factors influencing the risk of coronary artery disease have been discussed. It is easy to be overwhelmed by it all . The cynical view is 'everything is bad for you, so why bother?' So let us move on to a sharper view of what an ordinary, prudent person should do to reduce the risk of developing coronary artery disease.

What should an average person do to avoid heart disease?

First, he or she should remember that the seeds of coronary artery disease are planted decades before any symptoms appear. Even events in childhood could be important. Breastfeeding enthusiasts have tried to establish that bottlefed babies get more heart disease in later life. They have convinced most experts; but it is clear that any changes in 'lifestyle' have to be continued for many years if they are to be effective. The earlier they are started the greater the chances of success. This means that any changes must not be too arduous. He or she must be able to live with them.

Taken in this context a moderate change in diet sustained from early life may be better than a sudden drastic alteration in middle age when a friend or neighbour has a myocardial infarction. Everybody should reduce their fat intake and change some of the saturated, animal fat to polyunsaturated, vegetable fat. Routine measurement of the blood lipids is not required because everyone will benefit from this advice. Even people with 'normal' lipids can diminish their risk of heart disease by reducing their lipids still further. Blood tests will be required in those with a strong family history of raised lipids or with other medical reasons for suspecting that the concentrations may be grossly elevated. In addition food intake should be adjusted to prevent obesity.

Stopping smoking is the best manoeuvre of all. Its benefits start within a year, unlike most other risk factors. When you smoke a cigarette remember that your life is reduced by about the same time it takes you to smoke it.

Controlling an elevated blood pressure is also very important. Remember that hypertension rarely produces symptoms and the only way of finding it is to measure it. Many general practitioners will check their patients' pressures when they have the chance, but if you never give them the opportunity the raised pressure will be undetected until a stroke or heart attack occurs. Get it checked at least once every 2 years when you are over 35 years old. If tablets are required they should not produce side-effects. Go back to the doctor and ask for a change if necessary. Whatever type of treatment is decided upon, the pressure will have to be measured regularly for years to come.

The amount of exercise performed is a matter of personal choice. Nearly all of us could usefully increase it. But the exercise must be fun or it will become a misery. An old joke has some truth in it — 'Jogging may not make your life longer, but it certainly makes it feel longer'. Some people enjoy a daily run; others would do anything to avoid it. Incorporate the physical exertion into your daily routine or regular leisure activities. If possible, join in with other people. Stick with it, even if it is raining or you are in a hurry.

As we have seen earlier in this chapter stress and personality are controversial topics in the prevention of heart disease. Vague advice is often given to 'take it easy'. This instruction is not very effective. Overstriving people, who might benefit, ignore it, while others, who are already taking life fairly gently, do even less. It is very doubtful if personality can be changed and it is probably best not to try. If heart disease has already occurred, specific advice on 'lifestyle' may be needed, but that is another matter.

Should governments take more action?

Over the centuries the major priority of national governments has changed. Originally their purpose was to protect their citizens from external aggression or to provide that aggression. Later the correct religion seemed very important. Recently economic welfare has been of overwhelming significance. Other aspects of government are judged not only on their merits, but also on their economic costs.

Unfortunately, in the short term preventative medicine can clash with economic welfare. The reluctance of succesive British governments to do anything effective to reduce cigarette sales has already been referred to. It seems that the health of the tobacco industry and the health of the tax revenue are more important. Another example is a continuing attempt to promote the dairy industry, if necessary at the expense of increasing heart disease. Milk is a very good food for a young child or a malnourished adult.

But it is unlikely to have any special benefits for anybody else. Nevertheless the national consumption of milk products is maintained by a variety of subsidies to keep prices down.

Most doctors would like their governments to take more account of the health aspects of any policy decisions. In Britain this aspect is usually ignored unless firm public pressure has been applied. In the long term the voters have the final word. Once governments fear that they could lose elections by ignoring health issues the dominant role of economics will be modified.

Postscript

Realism is important in the prevention of heart disease. Nobody is perfect and good advice is often going to be ignored. Indeed the advice is often accepted by the wrong people. An overweight, heavy smoking, sedentary man will usually take little notice, while the person who is already taking reasonable precautions may drive himself to unnecessary perfection. Small changes that persist are better than drastic modifications that are soon dissipated.

Even the most dedicated probably think once in a while - is it worth it? Yes, it certainly is. The evidence is strong that the risk of coronary artery disease can be reduced; thousands of people are dying unnecessarily. But the immediate benefits of a healthier 'lifestyle' are also large. Giving up smoking, losing weight, and exercising more make you feel and look better. This alone makes it worth it.

We should also recall that we can reduce the incidence of coronary artery disease but we cannot yet abolish it. Nobody's life should be severely restricted for a goal that cannot be fully achieved. A large myocardial infarction which might have been prevented by few simple precautions is tragic. But a large infarction in a man who has forced himself to run in misery every night, who has not eaten strawberries and cream for years, and who has forgotton what an egg looks like, is even more tragic. Much heart disease can be avoided, but do keep a sense of proportion.

OK ?

The rest is up to you.

Selected reading list

Written for the General Public

E J Burke and J H L Humphreys (1982) *Fit to Exercise,* Pelham Books
  Practical advice on exercise
B Lewis (1980) *The Heart Book,* Barrie and Jenkins
  Emphasis on the benefits of diet
Risteard Mulcahy (1980) *Beat Heart Disease,* Martin Dunitz
  Emphasis on the benefits of exercise
E O'Brien and K O'Malley (1983) *High Blood Pressure,* Martin
Dunitz
  Good advice for those with this common condition
J P Shillingford (1981) *Coronary Heart Disease: The Facts,* Oxford
University Press
  Useful pocketsize book for patients with coronary heart disease
D Wainwright Evans and M A Greenfield (1978) *Cooking for Your
Hearts Content.* British Heart Foundation
  Many good recipes

Written for the Professional

G A Gresham (1976) *Reversing Atherosclerosis,* Charles C Thomas
  Thorough account of this major topic
S C Jordan (1979) *A Synopsis of Cardiology,* John Wright & Sons
  A basic textbook
D G Julian (1983) *Cardiology,* 4th Edition Ballière Tindall
  Good basic textbook
S Oram (1981) *Clinical Heart Disease,* 2nd Edition Heinemann
  Medical. A reference book
R S Winwood (1981) *Essentials of Clinical Diagnosis in Cardiology,*
  Edward Arnold
  Cardiology at the bedside

Index

blood lipids   47, 48, 61, 188—196
  risks of heart disease   51, 190—
  193
  reduction by diet   194, 195, 207,
  211
  reduction by drugs   195, 196
blood pressure   **see** hypertension
blood tests   32, 63
blue babies   116
bradycardia   133, 141—148
British civil servants study   199
bumetanide   84, 86
bundle of His   10, 131, 135
bundle of Kent   135
Burinex   **see** bumetanide

'cabbage' operation   164
caffeine   208
calcification of heart valves   95, 101
calcium antagonists   56, 59
cancer
  bowel   196
  heart   130
  lung   130, 179
  mouth and gullet   179
capillary   6
carbohydrates   203, 204
carbon dioxide   6, 158
carbon monoxide   179
cardiac biopsy   170
cardiac catheterization   36, 37, 56,
  66, 71, 105, 119, 122, 126, 165
cardiac massage   78—80
cardiomyopathy   82, 123, 170
cardioplegic solution   158, 160, 169
cardiopulmonary bypass   155—
  159, 160
cardioversion   141, 142
Carpentier-Edwards valve   162
catecholamines   76, 124, 176, 198,
  199
catheter   37, 39, 42, 43, 66
chest X-ray   22, 26, 35, 82, 101,
  119, 125, 127
cholesterol   **see** blood lipids
chordae tendinae   95, 96

chronic bronchitis   128, 129, 179
chylomicrons   187
cigar smoking   179, 180
circulation
  antenatal   111, 112
  pulmonary   6
  systemic   6, 158
  circus movement 134, 135, 143
clofibrate   195, 196
clot   **see** thrombosis
coarctation of the aorta   86, 115,
  158
coffee   206
conducting system   10, 11, 131,
  132, 142, 145
congenital heart disease   94, 108,
  109—123, 145
  cause 109, 110
  diagnosis   119, 120
  incidence   110
  surgery   121, 122, 161, 164
congestive cardiac failure   **see**
  heart failure
congestive cardiomyopathy   123,
  125, 126
connective tissue disease   97
contrast medium   38, 40
control of the heart   11
Cordarone X   **see** amiodarone
  Cordilox   **see** verapamil
coronary angioplasty   167, 168
coronary arteriogram   39, 56, 74
  162
coronary artery spasm   58
coronary artery vein grafting   56—
  58, 71, 74, 161, 162—164, 167
coronary care unit   42, 64—66, 72,
  75, 183
coronary sinus   10
coronary thrombosis   **see**
  myocardial infarction
cor pulmonale   128
crescendo angina   53
cyanosis   115, 116, 117, 118, 120,
  121, 122
cyclopenthiazide   86

216

valve
  aortic   6, 15, 49, 93, 97, 98, 100,
  104, 105, 107, 114, 130, 161, 166
  mitral   6, 35, 92, 96, 97, 98, 100,
  103, 107, 128, 161
  pulmonary   6, 92, 99, 114, 117,
  128
  tricuspid   6, 92, 97, 99, 100, 128,
  159
valve disease   82, 92—106
  catheterization for   37
  causes   93-98
  complications   102—104, 106—
  109
  surgery   105, 159
  treatment   104—106
valvotomy
  mitral   158
  pulmonary   114
variant angina   see atypical angina
vasodilator drugs   85, 86, 91, 104
vegetations   107
veins   8, 37, 162
  coronary sinus   10
  inferior vena cava   8, 38
  superior vena cava   8
  pulmonary   6
venesection   122, 123
venous pressure   20, 83, 100
ventilator   160, 165
ventricle   25, 112, 131
  left   6, 37, 83, 96, 124, 125, 126
  right   6, 37, 83, 117, 128, 148, 150,
  170
ventricular dilatation 97, 102, 129
ventricular fibrillation   65, 75—77,
  201, 207
ventricular septal defect   112, 117,
  120, 167
verapamil   56, 59, 125, 140,
very low density lipoproteins   189,
  190
  viruses   125, 126, 127

warfarin   70, 73, 104, 107, 162, 163,
  173
water softness   207

Wolff-Parkinson-White
  syndrome   135, 138

Xylocard   see   lignocaine